NORTH CAROLINA
STATE BOARD OF COMMUNITY C
LIBRARIES
ASHEVILLE-BUNCOMBE TECHNICAL COMMUNITY COLLEGE

S0-CUS-772

DISCARDED

JUL 2 5 2025

COLLEGES

DISCARDED

JUL 23 '85

BEYOND THE STREET

BEYOND
THE
STREET

A Handbook for EMS Leadership and Management

by

Joseph J. Fitch, Ph.D.
with
RICK KELLER, EMT-P, DOUG RAYNOR, PH.D and CHRIS ZALAR, RN

A J E M S B O O K

JEMS Publishing Co., Inc.
P.O. Box 1026, Solana Beach, CA 92075
(619) 481-1128

Editors:
  Keith Griffiths and Valla Howell

Book and Cover Design:
  L. Ortiz Art Services, (619) 232-3238

Book Publishing Consultant:
  Luster Industries, (619) 265-8171

Library of Congress No. 87-82161
ISBN 0-936174-04-8

Copyright©1988 by JEMS Publishing Co., Inc.

JEMS (Journal of Emergency Medical Services)
is published by:
  JEMS Publishing Co., Inc.
  P.O. Box 1026
  Solana Beach, CA 92075
  (619) 481-1128

All rights reserved. This book is protected by copyright.
No part of it may be reproduced in any manner or by any
means without written permission from the publisher
except by a reviewer who wishes to quote brief passages
in connection with a review written for inclusion in a
magazine, newspaper or electronic broadcast.

Printed and bound in the United States of America

6   5   4   3   2   1

To the EMS team members and leaders who have the courage to innovate, learn and grow.

Contents

Part I
EMS as a Team—Personnel Management

**Part II
Developing The Game Plan**

Part III
The Buck Starts Here!

Part IV
Calling The Plays—Operational Matters

Part V
Working With Other Teams:
Groups That Affect Success

Part VI
Appendices

Figures

Foreword

"The street" is what EMS is all about for most of us It's the challenging environment where the theory, the training and the preparation collide with people in every conceivable form of distress. After a few years of confronting and handling those emergencies on the street, most of us begin to ask what's beyond the street. Where will this career lead us?

The complex array of people, vehicles and other resources that are necessary to deliver prehospital emergency medical care must be organized and managed. Throughout the first 20 years of EMS, organization and management included a lot of stumbling, guesswork and trial-and-error. We were all learning—mostly from our own mistakes and those of others. Nobody with real-world experience seemed to have the time or the talent to construct a reliable framework for anticipating and skillfully handling the working environment of the EMS manager.

This book fills that gap. Those who question where their careers in EMS will lead them now have a tool for helping to design their own destinies. Jay Fitch and his associates have constructed the framework needed by those who strive to contribute to EMS "beyond the street."

Just a quick review of the table of contents reveals that this book deals with all the structural and financial issues of EMS. But it concentrates on the most important element—people. That emphasis reflects the fascinating career of the principal author.

When I first met Jay Fitch, he was a street medic and he was wondering where his career in EMS would lead him. Like so many of us, he was torn between that satisfaction of providing emergency care on the streets and the desire to influence the system at a higher level—beyond the streets.

Once he made the first big step into EMS management, Jay never looked back. Through diligent self-preparation and courageous acceptance of every-larger challenges, he became one of the best examples of upward mobility in the EMS field. In the process, the character of the man was apparent as he assumed the role of mentor, attracting young people with whom he shared his knowledge, skills and insight as they sought a career beyond the street.

Publication of this book is one of those landmark events that

eventually will affect many others. Many of the attitudes of the good
EMS manager are learned, and this book provides the structure and
the content for the needed learning. Already, before the book even
went to press, I have used the manuscript as a reference before going
into critical meetings. It is destined to be that kind of resource—dog-
eared and coffee-stained, ever present on the top of your desk.

Thinking back over all the EMS managers I've met, a common
theme strikes me as the difference between success and failure. It's
the same theme that runs throughout this book. EMS is a team process
and people are the most important commodity we have to work with.
They are fascinating in their differences and the infinite kinds of
challenges they can present to the manager.

As we share and learn from the insights of Jay Fitch and his
associates in this book, we should note that every aspect of the EMS
manager's job requires approval, attention, understanding and
cooperation from people both higher and lower on the career ladder.
In the management environment, system glitches can't be zapped into
rhythm, and non-conformists can't be restrained into conformity.
That's life beyond the street, and we are grateful to Jay Fitch for blazing
a clear and interesting trail through the wilderness of EMS
management issues.

—*James O. Page, J.D.*

Preface

Throughout this book we emphasize the importance of a "team effort." That's because we feel it's the *best* way to lead an EMS system. A team effort is consistent with current management principles—besides, it's more fun than doing it all yourself. This book is an example of our commitment to "walk the talk" as it was created through the collective efforts of those dedicated EMS professionals from throughout the country representing every facet of the industry. Members of our team who contributed significantly to this book include: Stephen Davis, Kate and Jim Dernocoeur, Judy Haffner, Richard Keller, Doug Raynor and Christine Zalar.

Dozens of ambulance services, EMS managers and fire and police officers provided us with information and insight. We sincerely thank all who contributed directly and indirectly for their willingness to share their experiences with us.

This book is not only designed to provide information, but to encourage managerial skills in the ambulance, fire department and emergency medical service systems. It may seem a bit theoretical at times, but in management, as in paramedic field-education programs, understanding theory is a must in order to apply the skills appropriately.

This book would not have been possible without the commitment to quality prehospital medical care by ambulance services—public, private and volunteer—and without the leadership and support of the State of Missouri's Department of Health and of the people in the Bureau of Emergency Medical Services.

A few final notes. Some argue that the use of the pronoun "he" is sexist writing. However, to avoid the clutter inherent in the awkward phrases "he or she," "him or her," "his or hers," I've chosen to use "he" throughout. I trust our female audience will forgive this as yet unsolved transgression in our English language and accept that, for now anyway, *he* also means *she*.

Throughout the book we use examples and case studies to give the theoretical discussions a more practical turn. In all instances, the names of organizations or people used in these examples are fictitious and should not be construed to represent actual individuals, places or events.

—*Jay Fitch*

1

EMS as a Team— Personnel Management

Is EMS A Team Sport?

Overview

Unequivocally—YES! Emergency medical services *is* a team sport. Good management of ambulance systems requires basic knowledge of the players involved, awareness of the rules of the game, and a know-how of team-coaching responsibilities. In addition, it involves learning to develop a winning game plan, financing the team, calling specific plays and working with other teams. The *goal* is saving lives. The *mission* is making a profit. Granted, public, private or volunteer services may define "profit" differently, but each group exists for a reason and therefore has a "profit" incentive. The profit may be expressed in either lives saved or dollars earned, but it should nevertheless be expressed. In this way, the benefit is measurable and gives purpose to the "game."

Effective management of EMS systems is complex. Until recently, this complexity and the critical need for competent leadership have been overlooked. Initially, federal dollars made it easier to play the game. With the passing of time and

(continued on next page)

(continued)

the elimination of this "free" money, many systems fell on hard times. Public and private systems alike went to their communities for increased subsidies. Because systems basked in both a positive image and favorable support generated by the TV show *Emergency*, for a short while this strategy was successful. Some systems were even upgraded to advanced life support. Somewhere over the years, however, the rules of the game changed. Taxpayer revolts, double-digit inflation, skyrocketing hospital costs and reductions in revenue-sharing dollars are just a few of the reasons for the changes. The coaches were dumbfounded! Prospective payments, DRGs, HMOs, PPOs, HCFA and a host of other players joined the league. Unfortunately, and with few exceptions, EMS managers remained asleep in the locker room while the game was being played. WAKE UP! It's now the seventh inning and the entire team depends on *you* to not only make a difference but to *lead* them to victory over death in the ditch.

The ideas presented here may seem radical to some, realistic to others. This book has been written to help you develop the tools necessary to get *results* as an EMS manager.

TEAMWORK

For organizational teamwork, one must hire, train and develop the right people for specific jobs in the organization. In addition, a manager is responsible for getting the staff to cooperate with one another and to coordinate its efforts in achieving the service's goals. The manager's job as motivator is never over. He must constantly strive for better team effort. Unless this is done, a manager will fail to reach top productivity despite the fact he may have the best people working for him. A group of individual all-stars without team effort will be beaten by a group of untalented people who have pulled together as a team.

Some years ago, it was thought that a manager was most effective when literally dictating to others what jobs had to be done and how to do them. Recently, however, we've learned that dictatorial methods don't work nearly as well. We've learned that team development, the giving and receiving of input and ideas from all team members—not just managers—is far more effective. To compete in the major leagues today, managers must understand, model and practice teamwork.

There are specific things a manager can do to inspire teamwork, but unless the basic climate and working conditions are right, the desired result won't be achieved. The key to teamwork is twofold: cooperation and the individual team member's desire to do a good job. To achieve this, a manager must ensure his employees' needs, both physical and psychological, are respected.

To develop teamwork, the manager must be a leader. He must treat people fairly and give them credit for work well-done. The leader must know the job. If he's incompetent, people will have little confidence. On the other hand, if he's competent people will respect him and won't object to a demanding approach. Generally, EMS personnel want to be identified with a successful operation, and they're quick to recognize a manager who can lead them to it.

The more people are drawn into the act by democratic or participative leadership, the more they'll feel a part of the team. It's the manager who must delegate responsibility and authority, then develop others to assume it. EMS personnel will respond positively to this trust placed in them. Important, also, is communicating to people what is expected of them and showing appreciation for a job well-done.

The conscientious ambulance service manager checks on those individual players not contributing to the team effort. He constantly evaluates each team member's effectiveness in achieving his personal goals and in cooperating with the organization as a whole. Outstanding patient care, patient *service* and team cooperation must be emphasized. The manager must not let people escape with sloppy work. Those who don't cooperate should be coached and counseled with sincere attempts made to improve poor attitudes and efforts. An individual unable to fit the group effort must be removed. If not, team spirit may be damaged or destroyed.

Good planning is also important in EMS teamwork. It's also a full-time job, involving the already discussed organizational and communication skills. Unless management plans ahead, it's difficult, if not impossible, to get the group functioning as a team. The manager must involve team members in this planning, communicate the final plans to the team and follow up to see that they're carried out.

This is the background required in any EMS situation. In addition, there are specific techniques required to develop teamwork. The best way to learn about teamwork is to look at the great teams in sports. Those who achieve seemingly effortless coordination do it by teamwork. The championship football team is an ideal example. In studying this professional team effort, we see that the most important thing in teamwork is having a purpose. The purpose in football, of course, is to win games. The greatest teams of all are those in which individuals are dedicated to winning the game and, in the process, forget about personal stardom.

In EMS, the teamwork achieved depends on the leader's ability to arouse organizational loyalties rather than personal loyalties. In the emergency medical service industry, as was noted earlier, the purpose or mission is to achieve efficiency, production and profit. This purpose is vital to the survival of any service, public or private. However, to get individuals really excited about their work, it's important managers understand that most people are attracted to this profession out of a genuine concern for others. Helping people in medical distress— even saving lives occasionally—is a high purpose! The greatest team effort in history happened during World War II. Why? Because there was a goal—an important goal. "Saving the world for democracy" was an ideal to which individuals dedicated their lives. They made unbelievable sacrifices. They went beyond the call of duty to achieve the larger purpose of *saving the world*—yet there was no *monetary profit for most of them.*

In both the EMS and medical-transport industry, our mission is equally important. Every manager must ensure that excellent service is provided, and the more the service aspects are spelled out, the easier it will be for the team members to grasp. What is the purpose of your emergency medical service business? What service does it render to the community? If this is clearly defined to employees, and if they believe they have an opportunity to contribute toward a goal, they'll be inspired to work together.

Humanitarian and profit-making purposes are the keys to teamwork. The manager's job, of course, is to keep the organization alive. He must keep the team constantly aware of its purposes and motivated to achieve them. If team members aren't constantly aware of organizational goals, they focus on small goals—those which may only advance their personal ambitions. They may put special effort into doing things on the job which give *them* satisfaction but which don't contribute to the overall achievement of the organization.

The only way to keep individuals from pursuing their own interests at the expense of the company is to clearly define the organization's purpose. The organization's mission statement is an attempt to express the purpose and philosophy of the company. For example, John Rester, president of Mobile Medic Ambulance Service, Gulfport, Mississippi, shares his mission statement: "The mission of Mobile Medic Ambulance Service is to provide the highest quality patient care that is cost effective to the communities we serve, while promoting individual and corporate growth and profitability."

Once the organization's purpose has been clearly defined in its mission statement and goals established, it's important to let people know how effective their contributions are toward the organization's original purposes. They need to know where they fit into the picture. They need to know that their manager recognizes their achievements.

For teamwork, it's important that everyone knows as much as possible about the overall operation of the organization. Each member should know the connection between his work and the work of others. He should know how the team is progressing and what the score is. It's a dull football game, indeed, when no score's kept. All of this serves to indicate the importance of telling people how they stand in achieving the goals and aims of the organization.

The manager must tell each employee the importance of his particular job and its relationship to the mission. Give him the big picture. People need to be reminded of their importance to the organization and that the entire organization's performance is linked to their performance. For example, you should emphasize how cleaning and stocking vehicles contributes to the final product of delivering high-quality patient-care services. It's not just the little job that counts, but the assistance to the total effort.

The person doing an outstanding job with paperwork is important. It's one of the most important communication links between the company and its customers. If invoices and statements aren't correct, money doesn't come in and the service can't operate. Base hitters make contributions to the game, but so do batboys! The more you can get people to feel excited about and to recognize the importance of their particular tasks, the more likely they are to stay with the team.

It's just as important that you listen to people so they can tell you how they're doing. A manager has a lot to tell the team, but the team also has a lot to tell the manager—if he's willing to listen. One of the best ways to encourage teamwork is to call conferences. Conferences encourage people to contribute and share ideas. What's the problem?

What can they do about it? Keep reminding them of their larger purpose and its relationship to the total organizational output. Anything that contributes to the total effort is cause to call people together for their ideas—this reminds them that they're on a team. Keep using team words by saying, "*we* are doing this," or "*we* are planning that." Convince them they can help the team by sharing their ideas.

Sometimes praise can be given in such a way that it involves a team effort. Praise a person for good work, but particularly praise him for his contributions to the overall goals of the organization. Specify *how* his contribution helped the organization meet its goal. Praise personnel in front of other workers so they will get the idea of teamwork, and encourage other people to join in and compliment each other for the good work that helped the organization reach its goals.

Do you have people in your employ who are sloppy and careless, whom you would not want to care for your family members, who do not do a thorough job? Or maybe you have some who chisel and take advantage of their position, who pass the buck and refuse to make decisions, who do what they're told but won't do anything beyond this or who won't help others with their work. If you have any of these problems, you have team problems. And the only way to solve them is to get people working as a team.

No matter how efficient each employee becomes, no matter how good your team gets, you will never achieve "perfect" teamwork. The only way the manager can hope to get anywhere near 100 percent performance is to keep coaching, instructing and guiding the team toward achieving the mission of the organization.

Leadership

Overview

What is leadership? Its qualities are difficult to define, but not nearly as difficult to identify.

Effective leaders don't *force* others to go along with them. Instead, they *bring* others along. Leaders get commitment from others by giving it themselves, by building an ambulance service that encourages creativity and by operating with honesty and fairness. EMS leaders demand much of others, but they also give much of themselves. They are ambitious, not only for themselves, but also for those who work with them. They seek to attract, retain and develop other people to their fullest potential.

Outstanding leaders aren't "lone rangers." They recognize that the organization's strategies for success require the combined talents and efforts of many. Leadership is the catalyst for transforming those talents into results. It's about getting people to give their best, leading people to their fullest potential and motivating them toward a common good. EMS leaders make the right things happen when they're supposed to.

An outstanding and effective EMS leader is someone who

(continued on next page)

(continued)

has respect. Respect is something you give in order to get. An EMS leader who has respect for others' work, abilities, aspirations and needs will find the respect they give is returned tenfold.

In theory, EMS managers are the coaches to a team effort in the truest sense of the word. EMS leaders are capable of independent thought and decision. They exude self-confidence and emotional stability. They bring order from chaos. They're sensitive to the needs and feelings of co-workers.

In practice, EMS managers help groups attain their own objectives by using the groups' fullest capabilities, while never losing sight of their own identities. They're a combination of the power vested in them by the organization as well as their own personality. They must be responsive to the needs of the organization. Leaders lose effectiveness if their decisions are either unacceptable to members of the group or if their authority is undermined. They have to demonstrate both personal fortitude and ability to motivate others to produce.

Some EMS leaders are charismatic. Their subordinates tend to associate and identify with them. It's their personal charm and magnetism that binds followers to them in a way that transcends the limits of formal authority and reason. A combination of qualities such as competence, character and personality helps shape a charismatic leader. If this doesn't sound like you, or your leader, read on....

To be a leader in the prehospital-care industry you need *determination* to persevere; *confidence* to lead; *energy* to work hard despite your many commitments to home and family; and *support* from family, friends, co-workers and professional associations.

Management skills are different from the medical or technical skills required for working on an ambulance. As one moves up in management, greater management skills and fewer technical skills are required. The road to the top is not straight and narrow. To be successful, the proficient manager needs specialized skills and competencies which must be learned and practiced repeatedly.

MANAGEMENT SKILLS

There are five main types of skills that the EMS manager must master: people skills, administrative skills, communications skills, political skills and personal attributes.

The most important, *people skills*, involves the ability to lead and influence people to accomplish the organization's goals. Outstanding managers are sensitive to the needs of their co-workers, and they tend to focus on the continued development of their subordinates, while fostering competence at all levels in the organization. Outstanding managers tend to be self-reliant, but they also depend on the good instincts of others.

Administrative skills involve organization and planning. Included in these skills are problem analysis to determine appropriate courses of action, critical decision making, the ability to control and monitor the organization's activities and appropriate task delegation to subordinates.

Communications skills involve the ability to listen and grasp what's really being said. It also means communicating with subordinates and superiors on an informal or relaxed basis—"getting along" with others. An effective manager must have solid writing skills to communicate both inside and outside the organization. Letters mailed with spelling and syntax errors are usually the object of office ridicule. The ability to speak publicly must also be developed. Finally, reading skills are crucial. Many managers are unable to grasp the full importance of their role because they refuse to read. They read well enough, but simply don't take the time to read material that would increase their job performance.

Political savvy is a critical factor that influences the success of every EMS leader. There are no classes or tests in political skills. If you don't develop this "sixth sense," however, you'll not survive as an EMS leader. Political savvy involves all of the leadership skills outlined in this chapter, plus an acute sense of timing for choosing the time and place to fight—as well as knowing when not to.

The EMS director for the Missouri Department of Health was recently asked to review the ingredients for political savvy. Ken Cole, who has served in this position for 10 years, said that in order to survive as a successful EMS leader, a person must also have an intimate knowledge of the bureaucracy within which he operates.

According to Cole, in order for an EMS leader to be effective, he must develop a sense of timing, presence and awareness of the facts.

Not using the existing network is a common failure for many leaders. Not every issue with a superior, bureaucrat or politician has to be confronted. There are many other people in the system who may have more credibility with or access to a particular person. These people can help the leader reach a more positive outcome in a given situation.

In our collective experiences with political folks, we discovered another required ingredient—timeliness. If you agree to complete a project within a certain amount of time, do so—or be prepared to suffer the consequences!

Personal attributes are the most obvious—and the toughest—skills to hone. The most important personal attributes that every EMS manager must have are honesty and integrity. Without these two, none of the others matter. They can only be acquired by daily effort. There are lots of excuses for not being honest in EMS management. Each will come back to haunt you at some time in your career. Two other necessary attributes include a high energy level and stamina. EMS is no place for slackers! And finally, managers must be decisive when necessary, identify strongly with management, resist stress and be flexible.

There's no perfect candidate for EMS management. Ideal managers understand their strengths and weaknesses and tend to compensate for the things they don't do well. Management-skill development is a life-long process. Outstanding managers and leaders are neither born nor promoted. Rather, their necessary skills and abilities are learned.

Minimum management competencies that must be developed are *analytical*, in order to identify, analyze and solve problems; *interpersonal*, in order to influence supervise and lead people; and *emotional*, to be stimulated by crisis rather than exhausted by it—to bear high levels of responsibility.

Ambulance service leadership is more effective if subordinates sense direction and a team spirit. The paths to such leadership include *preparation* (knowing the issues and remaining calm in difficult situations), *taking responsibility* (heading projects, making decisions, being accountable and delegating), *caring* (about patients, subordinates, colleagues and superiors) and *being creative* (taking risks and being innovative).

STYLES OF LEADERSHIP

Many leadership styles exist within EMS organizations across the nation. There is no single correct style. Many ambulance leaders tend to use autocratic or tell-and-do styles. Being an authoritarian who makes most of the decisions is easier than meaningfully involving individuals in the decision-making process. In the short run, it may be more effective. In the long run, however, these leaders are rarely successful. We advocate a mixture of the styles annotated below. An important key to effective leadership is learning which situation deserves which style.

Figure 1.1   Continuum of Leader Authority

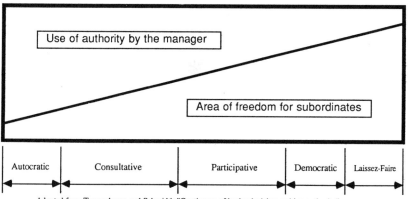

Adapted from Tannenbaum and Schmidt's "Continuum of leader decision-making authority"

Autocratic. In the continuum of leader authority presented in Figure 1.1, the autocratic end represents the manager who makes decisions and announces them to the group. Use of the tell-and-do style means that the manager has made a decision pertaining to the purpose of the group activity, how the group activity is to be structured and who is to be assigned to what specific tasks. The interactions and work setting have been decided by the manager. The role of the subordinates is to obey orders without altering the decisions already made. The manager provides little opportunity for a subordinate to participate in decision making.

In health-care settings, managers seldom use the autocratic style of leadership. It's often the older physician, in caring for patients, who develops this style. Out of habit, the physician may make decisions no one else can. Consequently, he or she makes them, announces them to other personnel such as paramedics and nurses, and expects them to be carried out immediately.

Consultative. The consultative style appears to the right of autocratic. In this situation, the manager may either *sell* decisions or present ideas inviting questions from subordinates. For example, he may say, "Tom, I think the 'rattletrap brand' ambulance is the one we ought to buy. It has everything we want on it and the price is right. What do you think?" In this style of leadership, the manager makes decisions concerning the job to be done, its purpose, how it's to be done, when and by whom. He then attempts to sell his subordinates on the decisions. He may recognize some resistance and invite questions. Unless overwhelming reasons are given, however, his decision is usually firm.

Participative. If a manager presents a tentative decision or problem to his subordinates, then gets suggestions and makes a final decision, we're dealing with a participative style. The manager identifies the purposes, problems and means of a job, presents a tentative decision, then seeks subordinate opinion ɔ make a final decision. In this instance, the area of decision freedom for subordinates is much greater and the use of authority by the manager is much smaller than with the autocratic and consultative styles.

The participative management style of leadership is a powerful motivator, enabling employees to have some influence and control over work-related activities. The work group influences decisions concerning work activities and their purposes.

Democratic. Within a democratic style the manager defines the limits of the situation, the problem to be solved, then asks the group to make decisions. As indicated in Figure 1.1 subordinates have a relatively large area within which to make decisions. Boundaries are set by the manager, who permits the group to make decisions within them. For example, an EMS supervisor assigns two paramedics to a unit, but permits them to decide who will give primary patient care and who will drive the unit, do the daily checklist, and so on. This style is fairly common in health-care settings.

Laissez-faire. The term laissez-faire originally meant that government shouldn't interfere with commerce. It's sometimes called free rein. Under such leadership, subordinates function within the limits set by the manager's own superior. The manager doesn't interfere with the group and participates in the decision-making process with the same influence as any other member of the group.

Subordinates have complete freedom in making decisions, with minimum participation by the manager. The manager is merely a figurehead. This style of leadership is rarely found in the administrative aspects of health-care organizations.

These variations only describe a manager's perception of his leadership qualities. Styles are not fixed. A manager should, therefore, focus on why he chose the style he did in a particular situation and on whether he made the best choice. No one style is always correct. For example, if a building is on fire, it's clearly not time for a participatory decision, even though the evacuation plan may have been a product of a group process. It's certainly more appropriate for the building manager to announce the decision to evacuate.

At this point, a good question to ask is "How does this relate to my ability to be consistent?" The answer is that similar situations should be handled the same way, no matter what style of leadership used. Even though styles aren't fixed, most managers have both a primary and a secondary style which they use most often. Think about the styles *you* use.

This section deserves careful attention and rereading. Concepts and practical applications of leadership and authority are often misunderstood by both EMS leaders and workers. It's difficult for medics to understand the wide diversity of decision-making styles within the organization. At one end of the continuum is the laissez-faire approach. For example, this style is used in the prehospital clinical setting when guidelines are established for treatment by medical control without day-to-day involvement of the administrative leadership of the service. In this situation, paramedics have freedom to use their own judgment within pre-established patient-care guidelines. On the other end of the continuum is an autocratic manager making decisions that may be politically necessary. For example, because the system is under financial scrutiny, the manager may decree there will be no "street drill" or cruising of districts between calls. Without an adequate explanation, this may seem oppressive to those who, until then, have enjoyed wide latitude of judgment in life and death situations. Failure to understand the dynamics inherent in rapid style changes, which may be necessary and appropriate to a situation, often wreaks havoc on the stability of the organization and the individuals involved.

Are you convinced management is not just "getting off the rig and taking it easy"? Ask this question: When you got out of EMT or paramedic school, were you good at what you did? If you're honest, you have to admit that experience and practice are a must for competency. The same principle applies to management. To be competent, you must repeatedly practice and learn from your mistakes. You must also recruit a winning team.

Personnel Recruitment, Selection and Orientation

Overview

There are several steps that will ease the entry of a new employee into the service. Whether the position is new or an established job that is being filled, care should be taken to recruit, interview, select and train the most appropriate person. These steps are illustrated in Figure 1.2. When one of these steps is rushed, personnel problems ensue. It's difficult and expensive for both the service and the employee to fire someone within weeks or months of the initial hiring because the manager didn't adequately do his job.

Recruiting personnel is an ongoing issue for most ambulance managers. Because of salary requirements and a young mobile work force, managers must constantly look for competent personnel. There are many options for developing an adequate pool of employees. When a position becomes available, either through the creation of a position or through attrition, several methods are available to solicit candidates.

(continued on next page)

Figure 1.2   Employee Selection and Orientation Process

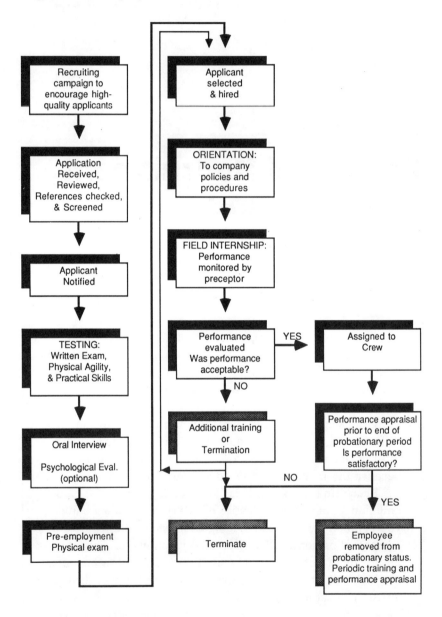

(continued)

First, current employees should be considered. Promotion from within is healthy for ambulance services, and the newly opened position becomes a lower-level job. In addition, the employee is not as threatening to the rest of the staff and is less of a liability to the service if there is unsatisfactory performance.

A second option in soliciting candidates is through area or regional EMT and paramedic training programs. Others advertise in those community newspapers that they know have good programs. Some organizations advertise in national trade journals. Many services rely on word-of-mouth or employee referrals.

No matter how you develop a pool of potential candidates, a systematic approach should be used to select them and to provide them with in-depth orientations. Such an approach *begins* with developing or reviewing job descriptions. One must know the job and performance expectations before either recruiting or considering applicants. Screening applications and resumes prevents spending time interviewing people who are not qualified.

Ideally, the selection process includes skill verification, physical and psychological assessment and an oral interview. The oral interview should be used to confirm the results of the other tests and to identify career objectives, job identification and social skills.

INTERVIEWING STRATEGIES

You've just lost a key dispatcher. Disgusted, and not sure what caused that person to leave, you're faced with another round of recruiting and interviewing to fill the position. It seems this endless business of hiring and re-hiring is like a merry-go-round. When does it stop? What's wrong with people anyway? What right do they have to leave us in a hole like this?

Sound familiar? Frustrating, to be sure. And expensive? You bet! It can cost as much as three times a key employee's annual salary to find a permanent replacement—or $45,000 to get another $18,000 dispatcher! What's worse, it's just possible that the continual hiring and re-hiring we often do for a single position may be entirely unnecessary.

What's the real problem? Inadequate attention to effective interviewing techniques is frequently why the right person isn't matched with the right job in the first place. Following are 10 do's and don't's which can make or break the effectiveness of an employment interview.

■ Do:

1. Plan ahead. Read the application thoroughly. Check background, education and references. Have a definite structure in mind, and on paper, for the interview. Then follow it.

2. Set a comfortable and open tone for the interview. Draw out the applicant in a relaxed manner, and encourage him or her to give you relevant data. "Stroke" the interviewee for pertinent information given and positive qualities presented. Reinforcement is a strong motivator and will lead the interviewee to offer more.

3. Remain non-judgmental and impartial throughout the interview. Observe, record and gather information— regardless of the data presented. You want neither to prejudge the candidate nor to reveal biases which may, from a Fair Employment Practices standpoint, border on the illegal.

4. Use either open-ended questions or reflective re-statement techniques, or both, in order to gain a maximum of information.

5. Before beginning the interview, clearly define the reasons for the interview, both your role and that of the interviewee.

6. Be specific about the position and the duties you expect the applicant to perform. Stay on track, and give all significant facts about the position and the organization.

7. Provide specific follow-up plans for the applicant, and for yourself, to follow as next steps in the employment process (for example, a tour of the facility, meetings with other key employees, tests to be taken and so on).

8. Arrange for a back-up interview, conducted by someone else,

to compare against your own perceptions and recommendations.

9. Include tests and other job-related assessment tools wherever practical.

10. Analyze the results of the interview. Rate the interviewee on a scale, using meaningful measures—and weigh this along with other information from tests, assessments, previous employment reports, other interviewers and raters to arrive at an informed and objective employment decision.

■ Don't:

1. Don't simply give the applicant's background a quick once over. Don't play the interview "by ear," or let it just "flow." Flowing is fine, but rambling wastes time and effort. Important data may be skipped.

2. Don't approach the interview as a Spanish Inquisition and demand information. Your applicant will likely respond to a hard-nosed approach with more of the same. And you'll gain little.

3. Don't question the applicant on matters which may be discriminatory on the basis of age, sex, race or religion. You're on safe ground only when your questions are job related. (This is a complex subject which requires a complete understanding of state and federal fair-employment statutes.)

4. Don't ask closed-ended questions which require only a yes or no answer. This only limits the applicant's responses.

5. Don't be vague about the reasons for the interview and your expectations of the person being interviewed. Don't generalize, wander off the topic or waste time discussing issues that are not relevant to the position or the applicant.

6. Don't ignore positive points and push ahead when opportunities for recognition or reinforcement present themselves.

7. Don't leave the interview without establishing specific steps to be taken—such as dates, times and the consequences of each for the applicant.

8. Don't rely solely on your own judgment regarding the applicant's suitability.

9. Don't use the interview only for a hiring decision.

10. Don't become a Freudian analyst or fixate on personality

traits. Instead, concentrate on the applicant's job-related qualities. Don't be more subjective than objective.

Many personnel specialists view the face-to-face interview as the *least* reliable way to select people for a job. Why? The possibility of human bias and just plain judgment error runs far higher than in other less subjective techniques such as test scores and performance assessment. If budget and time permit, the assessment approach, one in which several applicants are run through a series of simulated job-related performances, is more reliable.

For EMTs or paramedics, for example, a manager would ask an applicant to determine proper treatment in various simulated patient situations, to perform physical agility tests and to take detailed rescuer exams. The scored results would be compared with the scores of other applicants. Such a procedure would ensure that a candidate possesses the requisite knowledge and skills to perform the job well. Because these techniques are many times either too costly, time consuming or otherwise impractical for the small EMS provider, most managers continue to rely on the face-to-face interview as an employment determinant despite its less than ideal track record. After all, most say, it's just good common sense to sit down and talk with a person who's being considered for a job. No quarrel with that. But if the job interview is going to be "it," let's be sure as managers that *we* master the requisite skills and knowledge to do the task well.

USE OF REFERENCES

There are only two ways to handle references—thoroughly or not at all. To simply go through the names a candidate gives you is generally a waste of time.

If you decide to go the thorough route, Robert Half, in his book *How to Hire Smart,*† suggests the following:

Don't delay. Start checking references as soon as the candidate gives you permission to do so.

Ignore written references the candidate gives you. Written references some candidates carry with them to an interview are suspect for a couple of reasons. Letters written on the day of

† Crown Publishers, New York, N.Y., 1985.

termination are often written out of guilt. Sometimes such letters are written by the candidate himself.

Seek references the candidate doesn't mention. One way to do this is to call the candidate's previous employer and ask for somebody other than the person whose name you've been given. Another way is to ask a person whose name was supplied if they know another person you could talk to. Continue the pyramid until you've gathered enough information.

Call most former employers. A recent employer may not have bad things to say about a candidate, but that's not to say *previous* employers haven't had problems you'd like to hear about.

Get references by phone—not mail. People tend to be reluctant about *writing* negative remarks. Also when you're talking directly *to* someone, you're in a better position to judge his sincerity and enthusiasm about the person.

When filling a key position, make a personal visit to the person giving the reference. It's worth the time. People are usually more candid in a face-to-face situation than they might be over the phone.

EFFECTIVE ORIENTATION PROGRAMS

You've recruited, interviewed, checked references and chosen the best candidate to fill the position. And now it's time to begin the orientation process. Orientation is as important to both the ambulance service and the new employee as is the honeymoon to the newlyweds. It provides an opportunity to set the tone of the new relationship. That is, to develop feelings of mutual trust and to set firm expectations for excellent employee performance. This critical step is often overlooked or handled too informally. What happens in many ambulance organizations is that new employees are given their orientation by long-time employees, whose attitudes may need adjusting. Instead, new employees should be introduced by the best and brightest the organization has to offer.

For an orientation program to be effective, it should begin with an introduction to all key personnel. The new member should be made to feel a welcome part of a team effort. Once this is done, the following checklist will be helpful to ensure that a complete and effective orientation is carried out.

1. Complete all required W-4 and insurance forms.
2. Supply informational material including personnel manual, run reports, checklists and so on.
3. Supply company information such as its history, philosophy regarding patient care and innovations, structure, goals and objectives.
4. Review service delivery. This should include history; state, regional and local agencies; and components of the service delivery system.
5. Discuss medical control.
6. Discuss continuing education requirements.
7. Review daily activities. This should include the following:
     personnel manual
     standard-operating procedures
     employee-problems procedure
     field-complaint-resolution procedure
     job description
     paperwork
8. Review ambulance equipment.
9. Discuss lifting techniques.
10. Discuss communications procedures.
11. Review disaster plans.
12. Discuss special projects and committees.
13. Supply driving instruction.
14. Hold a field evaluation by a senior crew member.
15. Give a street test.
16. And, finally, conduct a performance appraisal.

Another important consideration in gaining and maintaining top performance is the degree of adequate *training* given to team members. This is covered in a later section.

Although nothing can guarantee employee performance, following these guidelines in the recruiment, selection and orientation processes can produce a higher quality staff member who is ready and willing to help the manager carry out the organization's goals and objectives.

The high costs of recruiting and orienting new employees have placed significant importance on programs designed to keep them within the ranks. Because of inadequate or non-existent retention programs, many ambulance services are suffering from employee turnover rates as high as 40 to 50 percent. The key element in retaining quality EMS employees is motivation.

Motivating Co-workers

Overview

One definition of motivation is "A 5-foot non-swimmer in 6 feet of water." A good manager must be a good motivator. He elicits the best from his people in order to accomplish the service's goals. While he directs and influences his people—in other words, motivates—a manager, at the same time, creates a climate in which the staff can find as much personal satisfaction as is possible.

Ambulance managers in rural systems complain that there aren't enough calls to get folks motivated. In urban programs, they've been heard to say, "Our staff is so busy running calls we can't get them motivated to do anything else." Urban or rural, motivation is a subject in which many EMS managers would receive low grades or an incomplete. There's a tremendous need and opportunity to link organizational goals to the employee's self-fulfillment. But the manager must understand the dynamics of the situation.

LINKING EMPLOYEE NEEDS
WITH ORGANIZATIONAL GOALS

Modern behavioral scientists tell us that people act or react in order to satisfy their needs. Unsatisfied needs cause people to behave a certain way in hopes of reducing tensions arising from these unmet needs. A person eats because hunger created the need for food. An EMT who has a strong need for achievement strives for advancement to a paramedic position. In other words, there is a reason for everything staff members do. One of the manager's responsibilities is to be sensitive to these tensions, or needs, that are present within each individual employee and to direct them creatively to the benefit of the organization.

Every person experiences different tensions. Some demand stronger and more immediate satisfaction than do others. Noted psychologist Abraham Maslow said motivation is based on a hierarchy of needs. Maslow's theory has gained wide acceptance over the years and helps us understand ambulance personnel's behavior today.

To understand Maslow's theory, picture a pyramid with five levels. (See Figure 1.3) The lowest order is *physiological needs* such as food, shelter, rest, recreation and so on. Normally, a paycheck enables a person to have the necessities and comforts of life that are vital to fulfilling these needs.

Figure 1.3   Level-of-Needs Model

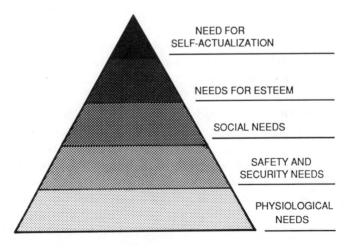

NEED FOR SELF-ACTUALIZATION

NEEDS FOR ESTEEM

SOCIAL NEEDS

SAFETY AND SECURITY NEEDS

PHYSIOLOGICAL NEEDS

When physiological needs are reasonably satisfied, needs at the next higher level begin to dominate and motivate the worker's behavior. These are usually referred to as *safety needs*. These we need in order to protect ourselves against danger and threat. We all desire more control over and protection from the uncertainties of life. In the ambulance service environment these uncertainties might be arbitrary management actions, loss of job, favoritism or discrimination. Most services have systems which meet these needs—systems such as personnel policy guidelines, provisions for medical benefits, unemployment compensation programs, and seniority are but a few.

Once the physiological and safety needs are met, *social needs* become important motivators of behavior. We need to belong, to associate, to feel accepted by co-workers, and we need to give and receive in friendship and love. Ambulance managers must be aware of these needs and to allow them to be fulfilled through informal groups within the organization. Tight-knit employee groups often threaten managers. They shouldn't. Informal groups can be powerful motivators.

Above social needs are the individual's ego needs for *esteem*, both self-esteem and esteem from others. Self-esteem includes a feeling of self-confidence, as well as a need for independence, achievement, competence and knowledge. These needs relate to the recognition of one's accomplishments, one's reputation, need for status and for appreciation. While prehospital care positions offer workers a high degree of satisfaction and appreciation, most of the recognition usually comes from patient contact rather than from a supportive management environment. As managers, we often miss the opportunity to stroke someone's ego. It's unfortunate because it's the cheapest benefit you can provide.

The highest level of needs is the need for *self-actualization*. This includes needs for self-fulfillment or for realizing one's own potential, for continued self-development or for creativity. Unlike the other four needs, self-actualization is seldom fully achieved. Most ambulance employees are struggling to satisfy their lower needs and divert most of their energy to satisfy them. Therefore, the need for self-fulfillment often remains unfulfilled.

So, you ask, how does this information help *me* manage? The answer lies in understanding each employee's level of need and then adapting your leadership style to help him meet that need. Many of the remaining sections in this book are designed to give you specific skills that will help you in that process. Most critical, however, is your attitude. Are you willing to work hard to motivate and encourage your co-workers so as to *assure* their success? If so, you'll assure your own success as well.

USING EFFECTIVE DELEGATION AS A MOTIVATOR

Delegation means transferring selected responsibility, along with commensurate authority, to one or more subordinates. Delegation means getting things done through others. To assure success and productivity in subordinates, a manager must take risks. He learns which team members are capable of doing which jobs by giving them the opportunity to try. In this way, delegation gives them the opportunity to practice success.

Top EMS managers often don't delegate well. All too often, managers give lip service to delegation and agree that it's essential, but then don't do it. Why? Managers' major fears include the fear of costly mistakes, a fear that subordinates might perform too well and show them up, a fear of losing control, a fear of losing prestige or status, a reluctance to give up an activity that they do well and finally, having no one to delegate to.

Following are five tips that will help managers delegate more effectively.

1. *Pinpoint functions to be delegated.* This means determining *what* responsibilities you can delegate, to *whom* they can be delegated and *how much* authority is to be given.

2. *Define standards and the objectives of the delegated responsibilities.* The subordinates should clearly understand the expected *results*, but shouldn't be told how to do the job. They should know already.

3. *Go slowly.* Depending on the subordinate, start with minor projects. It's easier for the manager to relinquish responsibilities by degrees, and the subordinate will be better able to absorb them and less inclined to feel overwhelmed.

4. *Consider the effect of delegation on the group.* If you select a subordinate to perform a certain task, how will the others view it? Will they feel that you're showing favoritism? Will they feel that you don't have sufficient trust in them or that you're asking one of the group to do something that you should be doing? Will they feel your

decision to be a good one and that it reflects your continuing confidence in them?

5. *Create short-term delegations.* This permits you to test more subordinates in a variety of assignments with least risk. It also gives you a better idea of individual abilities and capabilities.

For an EMS manager, the benefits of effective delegation far outweigh the risks. The primary benefit is that your time is spent on more important jobs. Other benefits include a better perspective, development of more competent subordinates, better communication, increased employee commitment and ultimately subordinates with greater confidence in their own abilities.

In the final analysis, delegation is a matter of trust and good business sense. If a manager understands that no matter how skilled he or she may be, accomplishments can be multiplied if subordinates are allowed to do the things that *they can* do. If allowed to make the decisions that *they can* make and to solve the problems that *they can* solve both subordinate and manager emerge winners.

CAREER-DEVELOPMENT OPTIONS

The patient-transportation industry is demanding, both emotionally and physically. Some say it's a young person's game. Odd schedules, stress and physical demands make it so. Few individuals ever spend an entire career with, and retire from, an ambulance service. This has had serious effects on the industry and the individuals that have chosen it for their career. State health officials have long been concerned with the attrition rate of field personnel. Some areas report that 60 percent of those licensed don't relicense after three years. This is due in part to the mobility of the work force and the youth of medics. It's cause for concern, however, when one considers that states subsidize training costs and that a chronic problem of inexperienced medics plagues services resulting in high turnover rates.

Does this mean that emergency medical services is a poor vocational choice? Not necessarily. For many, the real-world experience they gain provides them the opportunity for personal growth as well as a necessary stepping-stone to another career. A prehospital-care provider can see humanity at its very best—and at its very worst. If the person can avoid the stress associated with a lights-and-siren lifestyle, a career in EMS can be both fulfilling and rewarding.

Experts have found that most people entering this field do so out of a sincere desire to help others. This high purpose seems to wear off as prehospital-care providers forget that they work for an emergency medical or ambulance *service*. If they no longer desire or are no longer capable of providing highly personalized medical care and emotional support to *every* patient, it's time to consider another career.

Unfortunately, many paramedics and EMTs don't realize when this hardening process occurs and that their attitudes and lives are changing. Without early recognition, they leave the team feeling like losers.

What are the implications of this information for the effective EMS manager? The manager must recognize what's happening and develop strategies to prevent either a personal crisis for the employee or a general crisis for the service. How many years can a field person expect to effectively serve? What career opportunities are there? What can the manager do to avoid a crisis?

Career pathways for field personnel are narrow. On the technical side, they can progress from EMTs to paramedics, but then technical growth is limited unless they leave prehospital care. There are limited supervisory and training positions available. There are even fewer top-management positions, and many of these require advanced academic preparation. It's understandable why many field personnel feel trapped and, consequently, *un*motivated.

The question, then, becomes this: Should managers encourage personnel to build a career within the industry or to build a career through their experience in the industry? The latter is the only reasonable option. Career building can be accomplished in a variety of ways. Making sure new employees understand the situation can be strong motivation for them to continue in school or to make other plans for their long-term future. Tuition-assistance plans, short-term assignments within other departments, specialized employee counseling and career-development programs are but a few of the programs that have received wide acclaim in recent years.

A manager should help an employee develop his career plans, in writing, and should assist him in achieving those goals. There should be a regular informal review of his progress toward his personal goals. One manager called four EMTs into his office one day and said, "You guys are too bright to be working as street medics. Three years from today none of you are going to work here." While the employees were picking themselves up off the floor, the manager went on, "Figure out what you want to do, and then come back and tell me what I can do to help you do it." Although this shock treatment is not necessarily recommended, it did work. Five years later, three of the four were managers of large urban EMS systems. The fourth employee was still there, happily working as a competent field EMT. The moral to this true story is that it's the manager's responsibility to encourage his people to grow and then to support them, as individuals, no matter what choice they make.

C A S E   S T U D Y   # 1

Effective Delegation As A Motivator

Charlie has been a field supervisor for over a year. His EMT background goes back another two years. He's viewed as a pretty good supervisor, although he has indicated he wants to leave field operations eventually and get into management. Lately, he's been hanging around the dispatch board a lot, and the operations manager has overheard complaints from his crew about some conflicts they've had with him. John, the operations manager, feels he needs to talk with Charlie about these problems. John knows that Charlie has heard that the service may soon be hiring an assistant operations manager, but John doesn't feel that Charlie has what it takes to do this job. John's pleased, though, that Charlie has been taking some management courses on his own.

When Charlie's called in, John notices that he seems pleased at the opportunity to speak with his boss. But as soon as John begins talking about the problems concerning Charlie's spending too much time in dispatch and not enough dealing with his crew, his mood changes to discouragement and silence.

Here's a classic example of a good employee, discouraged because he sees no chance for further growth in the organization. Charlie feels frustrated and without further challenges on the job he may leave. What's John to do?

John knows that it's too soon to make Charlie his assistant. But it's clear that he needs and wants new challenges.

As John talks, he learns why Charlie has been hanging around dispatch. He wants to learn more about this area. And the frustrations he's been feeling have resulted in his conflicts with the crew.

The solution suddenly becomes clear to John. Because the service is soon to change over to system-status management, John has been asked to study this change and make recommendations. John can use help with this. Why not delegate a portion of this study to Charlie? Charlie's obviously delighted at the chance. He sees it as a way to make his views known and to gain a measure of recognition within the organization.

Delegating this work to Charlie is of value in many ways:

—He becomes a more motivated employee. He's being given a chance to practice success.

—John will have additional help on the project. Although it involves some risk, due to Charlie's inexperience in this area, he has demonstrated initiative to learn. There may be other people as well that John can motivate in this way—perhaps through the formation of a task force.

—The study will be completed in a shorter time with Charlie's help—an obvious plus to management.

This example illustrates a solution to a problem faced by many EMS managers: How to motivate employees given a limited degree of areas in which added delegation and responsibility can be given. Task forces or think tanks are an ideal means of creating valuable experience for staff—and at the same time providing a means for increasing motivation and enthusiasm. Since task forces often have a short time span, they create opportunities to test the success of delegated responsibilities and to form the basis for future decisions.

■   ■   ■

Communicating with Others

Overview

Once basic needs are recognized, it's important to develop a climate in which these needs can be addressed. Openness and trust are major factors in building the bridge to high-employee performance. Unfortunately, the way managers and supervisors usually communicate tears at the very foundation of this bridge. Because ambulance management is crisis-oriented and must operate in a decentralized environment, we often don't interact routinely unless there *is* a problem. This can create a climate that is defensive rather than accepting. Figure 1.4 outlines the types of behaviors and responses that can be used by a manager.

Communication skills include informal or interpersonal skills, oral and presentation skills, skills in writing and skills in reading. All of these, except reading, are influenced by the communication climate developed by a manager.

Figure 1.4   Developing a Climate for Effective Communication

The climate of a service affects the ability of members to work well together. One way to conceptualize the influence of climate is diagrammed below:

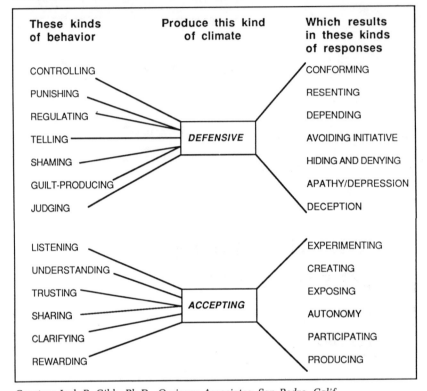

Courtesy Jack R. Gibb, Ph.D., Omicron Associates, San Pedro, Calif.

INTERPERSONAL SKILLS

Human communication is a social process. We act, react and interact. Direct communication breeds success in ambulance management. To communicate more directly, we identify and open the filters that operate when we communicate. Filters can be internal, external or environmental. Internal filters are feelings and thoughts. Prejudice is an example of an internal filter that can distort communication. External filters include specific behaviors such as actions or words. Environmental filters include the time and place of an interaction. Figure 1.5 outlines these filters.

Watching for visible signs of external filters has been popularized by many books on interpreting body language. Through simple

Figure 1.5 Environmental Filters

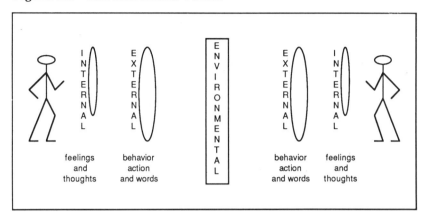

observation, a person can learn a great deal about what another is thinking and feeling. Someone once described this as *"Your words tell me yes, but there's no in your eyes!"*

Listening with both your eyes and ears is the key to effective employee communication—commonly referred to as behavioral communication. Recognizing and monitoring behaviors as well as their underlying motivations are important managerial skills. For example, at the end of a shift you observe a supervisor counseling an employee in the communications center. The employee has forgotten a small item on a run report and you hear the supervisor say he can't stand this person. The employee asks him why he's so angry. The supervisor says he's not angry but with such icy control that there's no doubt in the employee's mind that he's furious. What filters are operating in this interaction? All of them. Therefore, the mixed message the manager conveys blocks all productive manager-employee communication.

The internal filter is the supervisor's personal feelings about the person. The icy tone is a behavior filter. The fact that the interaction happened in the communications center at the end of the person's shift is an environmental factor which will affect the outcome of the interaction. Managers must choose the appropriate time to interact negatively or positively with employees. The end of a busy 24-hour shift is *not* the time to discuss a minor paperwork problem. In the previous example, the employee's fatigue affected the interaction, as did the fact that the meeting was held in front of others. The employee's self-esteem was at stake, creating additional tension. The supervisor did not improve performance because he failed to recognize the factors necessary for effective communication.

TECHNIQUES FOR EFFECTIVE LISTENING

There are several techniques at an EMS manager's or supervisor's disposal to reduce filters and improve listening skills. *The following will help communicate attentiveness* to the speaker. Face the individual and establish eye contact. Minimize external distractions while demonstrating positive body language. Then ask for examples, using short phrases to let them know to go on such as "mmmm," "I see," "Really" and "Oh."

In addition, there are four minimal responses that will improve manager-employee communications—clarify, paraphrase, reflect feelings and summarize. Figure 1.6 outlines examples of each technique and illustrates when they may be useful.

FEEDBACK

One of a manager's greatest assets in order to communicate effectively is the ability to give and receive feedback about a person's *behavior.* Feedback can be positive or negative. The goal in providing feedback in the work setting is to improve the other person's work performance. The following criteria should be evaluated when preparing to give an employee feedback, whether it be positive or negative.

Specificity. Feedback should be specific rather than general. To be told "your patient care is poor" will not be as useful as being told "the splint is not properly set."

Appropriateness. Feedback must meet the needs of both sender (the organization) and receiver (the employee). It can be destructive if it only serves the organization's needs, ignoring the employee's needs.

Usability. It should be directed toward behavior that the employee can change. Frustration results when a person is reminded about a shortcoming over which he has no control. For example, telling an EMT that he stutters when he talks with patients is unproductive and destructive if the employee can't control it.

Request. Feedback is most effective if solicited rather than imposed. Developing a trusting climate, as discussed earlier, encourages individuals to request feedback.

Timing. Feedback must be well-timed. In general, it's most useful when given soon after the observed behavior. Providing someone

Figure 1.6   Active-Listening Techniques

Type	Purpose	Examples
Ask for CLARIFICATION	To get additional facts or opinions.	Can you clarify this?
	To help explore all sides of an issue.	How do you think that occurred?
	To define a term	What do you mean by...?
	To encourage the speaker to analyze other aspects and discuss them with you.	Does that mean...?
PARAPHRASE for meaning	To check your interpretation with the speaker's intended meaning	As I understand it then, you mean...
	To show you understand what the speaker is saying.	Am I right, then, that you are saying...?
	To check your expectations of the speaker's behavioral intentions.	This is what you have decided to do and the reasons are...?
CHECK PERCEPTIONS for feelings	To show that you understand how the speaker feels at this moment	I imagine you feel pretty annoyed right now...
	To check the accuracy of your perception of emotion in the speaker.	You look pleased... You seem angry about what happened...
	To help the speaker evaluate and temper his or her feelings.	You seem a bit nervous. How can I help?
Make SUMMARIZING statements	To bring the discussion into focus.	As I have heard them, these are the key ideas you have mentioned...
	To serve as a springboard for further discussion.	So your main points are, then,...
	To check the overall accuracy of your understanding and for important points overlooked or left out.	Let me see if I can summarize what you have said...

Adapted from Federal Emergency Management Agency's "Basic Skills in Effective Communication" 1983 feedback on his behavior with a patient that occurred several weeks ago is often worse than no feedback at all.

Clarity. Check to ensure that filters don't block feedback. For example, have the employee paraphrase the received feedback to see if it corresponds with what was said.

When giving feedback, focus on the employee's *behavior—not* on the total person. A manager must separate specific behavior ("It doesn't look like you washed the rig.") from demeaning general criticism ("You are just never going to learn.") in order for his feedback to be heard and accepted.

Two final suggestions on feedback. Give it in a way that will help the employee improve his behavior, and praise whenever possible. A good rule of thumb is to give two doses of praise for every criticism. If you're thinking "I can't do that," then you're not doing your job. Go out and catch your staff doing something right!

USING OPPOSITION CREATIVELY

Most successful managers have had to overcome opposition to ideas they've introduced. Generally, employees will respond one of two ways to new ideas. One type of response supports and affirms the manager. "What you said is a great idea." The other type of response opposes and resists. "Boss, can't you see how wrong you are?" Support and opposition are very real forces in EMS life, and each can be used or wasted. Most people have some investment in their own ideas. For example, they may have taken a great deal of time and energy to develop an idea, and because of this they have strong feelings about it. When his idea is attacked, he may feel personally attacked. In extreme cases, he may feel great hostility. The result is that those who strongly challenge the idea may be mistakenly seen as the enemy when, in fact, they may be a potential friend and supporter. This is true no matter who presents the idea.

Managers can choose to resist, avoid or *use* opposition to their ideas. Traditionally, most EMS managers resist it. They obey Newton's law by meeting every force with an equal but opposing force. Therefore, they meet hostility with hostility, anger with anger. Other managers avoid or deny opposition. They ignore what other team members say or insist that "we're all really saying the same thing." This denial approach is like skating on thin ice. Eventually, when enough weight is applied, the ice breaks and the supervisor sinks.

A more constructive approach is to creatively use opposition. Opposition can be viewed as an opportunity to review, rethink and re-evaluate. For example, when an EMT is in an unfamiliar area, a map helps guide him in the right direction by the quickest possible route. In dealing with management ideas, plans and programs, it's helpful to consider opposition as guidance. Opposition can be the map which guides the manager toward preset goals in the most effective way.

To use opposition creatively, it's essential to turn *toward* the person with the opposing view. In doing so, there are several considerations. Analyze and identify the underlying causes of the tension. Create a climate in which opposition can be freely aired, thoroughly discussed and clearly evaluated. Be sure that all opposing views are understood by everyone participating. At this time, dialogue, not argument, is necessary. Realize that hostility and interpersonal conflicts may be expressed or suppressed. This is the time to use your creative listening skills, and remember, it's the idea being attacked, not the person.

A good manager will integrate the strong points of the opponent's ideas into the plan or program. He'll work to decrease the negative consequences of the conflict and recognize that opposing preferences may still persist. This is done by acknowledging each person's common goals, by appreciating the similarities in their ideas and by expressing warmth and respect for the other person. This last step is of *critical* importance. Even if an employee doesn't agree with the manager, but perceives that the manager has listened and respects him as a person, he's much more inclined to support the manager's idea or program.

In summary, to use opposition creatively first show that you respect the other person. Realize that you oppose the idea, not the person. Be open and honest in discussing the opposition, and allow honest feelings to be expressed. Listen to what's being said and then work to decrease the negative consequence of the conflict. Remember, everyone's working toward the same goal.

ORAL AND PRESENTATION SKILLS

There's a direct relationship between interpersonal communication and public speaking. An audience is simply a collection of people. The same principles of communication apply whether you're speaking to one person or to 100.

Be in control of what you say and how you say it. Understand your audience. Know how to use your voice and body language. Acknowledge your attitudes toward other people—in other words, know yourself. Use a personal speaking style that, although not perfect, shows you're an energetic, involved, direct and open person. And finally, understand your speaking situation and the limitations of the physical environment in which you're speaking.

In today's society, EMS managers must also understand that if they're to educate, they must reach out. Fifty years ago, people were content to listen to someone read a manuscript from behind a lectern. Today, in large part because of television, an effective public speaker must also stimulate or entertain if he's to keep his audience's attention. Following are four suggestions on how a speaker can be more effective.

1. Analyzing the target audience in preparation for a presentation is a step that can't be overlooked. Will the groups be large or small? Their age, sex, educational background, income level, religious and political affiliations and their reasons for attending the presentation are all factors which must be considered. Know your audience!

2. The structure of the presentation will have an effect on how it's received. The manager should prepare an outline, introduction, speech and conclusion.

3. The introduction builds common ground with the audience. It's their first impression of the speaker so it's important to establish eye contact and arouse curiosity. Effective speakers often begin their presentations with a dramatic or startling statement, with an anecdote or with a brief quote. Do what's natural.

4. The body of the speech contains your main points. (For example, that the Criss Cross Ambulance Service is worthy of the Rotary Club's support for a new defibrillator.) Remember, your audience has a limited attention span. Don't throw in war stories unless they support your main theme. It's wise to choose a framework within which you can comfortably organize your material. Following are some suggested frameworks.

Chronological analysis is effective for topics that can be explained by a time frame. This is well suited for informative presentations such as the history of EMS in "Criss Cross."

Inductive reasoning (arguing from specific examples to a general theme) is effective for persuasive speeches such as "lives are being saved by paramedics in Goodwill, and they will also save lives in Criss Cross."

Problem-cause-solution is also an effective strategy for persuasive speeches. Is there a serious problem? Is the proposed solution practical? Will the proposed solution solve the problem?

Deductive reasoning, beginning with a generalization and drawing a specific conclusion, is more useful in an emotional appeal than in a logical argument. For example, Goodwill has new ambulances, so we should too!

Analogy is an effective tool that works much like an anecdote. An analogy paints a vivid picture which helps the listener remember the speaker's point. "Investing in the community's ambulance service is like putting money in the bank. When you need it, you want the peace of mind to know it will be there."

The conclusion is as important as the opening. It should be strong and help listeners recall the presentation. Effective techniques include repeating a rhetorical question used in the introduction, especially if it's personalized ("How much is the life of your child or loved one worth?"), summarizing in a brief emphatic manner, inducing the audience to act ("Won't you please help us fight death in the ditch?), and predicting the future ("If we continue to neglect our responsibility to this program . . ."). These tools, if used appropriately, will give you a strong closing.

Finally, a few random thoughts about presentations. Use colorful visual aids to help illustrate, amplify or explain your topic. Be conscious of body language during your presentation. Stage fright is normal, and actually a little tension improves your performance. Remember, you don't have to be perfect. The key is to recognize that the unexpected may happen and to handle it calmly. Focus on the thought that you *know* your subject matter and that you planned and rehearsed your speech throughly. Practice in front of a mirror, your spouse, a friend or with a tape or video recorder.

WRITING SKILLS

Most EMS managers don't have the opportunity or time to make personal presentations to every person they'd like to. This is why writing skills are important. Many of the strategies used in oral presentations also apply to written communications.

Before writing the report, consider *to whom* am I writing and *for what purpose* am I writing? Don't delay in writing the report. Knuckle down, face reality and get to it!

Establish the report's objective. Determine *why* the report is being written. To inform? To persuade? Make sure that you and the person requesting the report agree on its intention. If your report is unsolicited, the full reponsibility for establishing its objective is yours.

An EMS manager's reading audience will most likely be a highly select and definable one. His readers will have a fairly narrow, technical, financial or professional interest and their needs will be directly related by their common profession. In order to best reach his audience, a manager should ask himself what information is necessary, what is the readers' knowledge of the subject, what are their attitudes. Recognize the readers' priorities through their various backgrounds, interests, needs, convictions and environments, then adapt your report to meet them. And while doing these things, never be condescending or arrogant.

Following are some do's and don't's in writing. First, the do's. Begin by outlining what you'd like to say in your report. By doing this, you'll not only eliminate unnecessary information *before* writing your report, but perhaps think of important data you would have otherwise neglected to include. (It's called brainstorming.) OK, you've finished your outline. Now start writing, using short declarative sentences–short and simple is your goal. A positive and authoritative voice, as well as accuracy, lends credence to your writing. Accuracy throughout is crucial, particularly with math. But *any* inaccuracy can destroy your reader's faith in whatever else you say. "If this guy doesn't even know this," they might think, "how do I know this is right?" They must feel good about what they're reading and feel confidence in what you're saying. Finally, show alternatives and their possible results, and explain any shortcomings in the report.

What to avoid? Don't make your report too long. Say what you have to say and leave. If you embark on an example, an explanation, or an illustration, get to the point–without too much distracting detail. Don't attach conclusions and recommendations to the wrong point. Make sure your conclusion supports your original thesis and clearly conveys your idea to those who must act upon it.

Just as important as writing style is the format of your report–particularly if it's long. In a long report, a summary is used to refresh the reader's varying interests. The summary contains four basic elements.

Purpose. The purpose should immediately reveal the subject's significance and the implications of the information.

Scope. This covers the information's relevance and the validity of the results. It defines limits and boundaries to eliminate misconceptions and unnecessary questions.

Findings or conclusions.

Recommendations. Briefly review the pertinent facts to ensure that the reader understands the issue. He'll then be in a better position to make an informed decision.

READING SKILLS

These skills, although self-explanatory, are often overlooked by EMS managers. This doesn't refer to a manager's ability to read as much as it refers to his *desire* to read that material which will make him more competent in his position. It's astonishing to see how many EMS managers have no idea of how to research what they need to know. Give yourself a pat on the back—if you've read this far, you couldn't possibly be one of those people, right? Successful EMS managers tend to read a lot, keep detailed files about all kinds of things and have an insatiable curiosity about ways to improve themselves and the service they manage. Remember, information *is* power, and everything you read—newspapers, professional journals or magazines—make you more aware of the factors and events that could be a threat or an opportunity to your service.

Changing On-The-Job Behavior Through Training

Overview

Ever hear of a major-league baseball team not going through spring training to prepare for the upcoming season? Training paves the way for improved team performance—in EMS as well as in baseball! Of course, it's not just spring training we're talking about here, but training every season of the year—month in, month out.

Why training? Let's put it this way. We've previously discussed management essentials such as good leadership, communication, delegation and motivation. But, as important as these skills are, they alone aren't enough to guarantee good team-member performance. Employees still need the knowledge, skills and techniques to do their jobs well. If they haven't received adequate on-the-job or formal training in *how* to do their jobs well, they'll turn in a disappointing performance, even with the best management skills in the world.

TRAINING—THE PROCESS, THE OBJECTIVES

What is training? Training is an ongoing process. It gives people the necessary knowledge, skills, techniques and attitudes that help them perform assigned tasks according to expected standards.

Training takes many forms—formal classroom instruction, practical on-the-job training from an experienced performer, periodic short courses, exposure to jobs other than the ones primarily assigned, training through TV or audio tapes and home-study courses. The point is, whatever form the training takes, the objective is the same—*to change or improve behavior on the job, behavior which can be seen, measured and evaluated.*

Let's look at some specific objectives that training addresses:

Increased productivity

Improved quality of work

Higher morale

Improved team cooperation

New skills development

Increased knowledge and understanding

Changed attitudes and perceptions

New methods, policies and procedures

New services or equipment (for example, data processing)

Preparation of people for job advancements or new positions

Reduction of wastes, costs, losses, turnovers, absenteeisms, and so on

Preparation of people for organizational changes (for example, expansion, merger)

Increased employee motivation and involvement

Knowing some of what training can address, let's look at *how* the training process works. Training, like communication, is a cyclical process. It generally starts with an analysis of the needs for training, and continues through planning, implementation and evaluation. The diagram in Figure 1.7 shows how this works.

Now for a closer look at each step of the cycle.

Figure 1.7   The Training Process—A Continuous Cycle

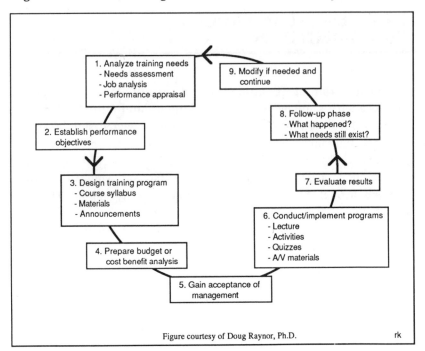

Figure courtesy of Doug Raynor, Ph.D.   rk

■ Step 1. Analyze training needs

This is not as simple as it seems. Sometimes, when a problem arises, we assume that training can fix it. For example, let's say the service is experiencing poor response times. The operations manager says, "Let's get to work on this. It's obvious the EMTs are goofing off, so we'll get them into a motivational training session and get ourselves up to speed." Sound reasonable? Only if the *real* problem is unmotivated paramedics. It's possible something else might be wrong. For example, hard-to-start poorly maintained vehicles could be wasting those precious moments, rather than the folks who operate them. Therefore, a thorough analysis of the problem will provide a clearer picture of what's needed.

Various techniques can be used to determine where the need for training lies. Some of these techniques include assessment through interviews and questionnaires, observation of on-the-job performance, performance appraisals and attitude surveys. Often, EMS services call in experienced consultants to assist in determining these needs which can then be met through training.

Of course, many needs within the EMS system can be clearly identified without all this fancy analysis. True enough, and if you're in that situation, go to step 2.

■ Step 2. Establish performance objectives

This is a vital step all too often overlooked. What exactly do we want to accomplish through training? In other words, to what standards do we want performance measured? Where is it now? Where do we want it to be? Performance standards are the stuff of which successful EMS outfits are made. It's OK to have a general idea of where we want to go. But, if *everyone* on the service team doesn't have a particular set of standards, spelling out what each person's performance is supposed to look like, we'll have a hard time getting where we want to be. So, when deciding upon changing behavior through training, know what those changes should be.

The standards which we expect people to follow are most helpful when they are integral to each person's job description. That way, both the employee and the supervisor, who will have to appraise the person's performance from time to time, have a clear idea of what that particular job entails. By establishing clear standards, a manager is better able to fairly appraise an employee's performance and judge if he's working at, below or above the set standards. For example, say you're hiring a dispatcher. The dispatcher's job description has been carefully written and includes some very specific performance standards. Among other things, the description says:

> 3a. Telephone call response. The dispatcher will quickly answer each call made to the service, and respond according to established protocol.
> *Expected Response Time:* 5 seconds, or less, on 90% of the calls.

Now, whether or not you agree with the standard, at least there's a specific guideline for phone responses. With proper logging and occasional spot checks, it'll be easier to appraise the dispatcher's performance standard.

Back to the subject of training. Let's say the data that's been collected indicates dispatchers have generally fallen on average to seven or eight seconds for phone responses. Obviously, this affects overall service-response time. You rightly determine that training is necessary to bring dispatchers back to a more acceptable level. Establishing a performance objective for this training program should be a breeze—to re-establish a standard phone response time of five seconds or less.

However, finding standards upon which to base performance objectives can be difficult. One good source is the U.S. Department of Transportation's Curriculum Guidelines. Both EMT and EMT-P curriculums define clear standards. Another source of information is state or local protocols. These establish standards by which your service's personnel can be measured.

■ Step 3. Design a training program.

Once performance objectives are established, it's time to decide the type of training which will best eliminate the problem. For starters, set up a course outline or syllabus, decide what training materials will be needed, determine how the training will be conducted (with lectures, films, discussion, case studies, etc.) and decide who will do it. Planning pays off! Is there someone on staff who's experienced in conducting a training session? How long should the training last? Will only dispatchers be involved, or should others attend as well? How will coverage be arranged when dispatchers are in training? Will the training be conducted during business hours or on free time? The questions are numerous and the options many. Some experience in both adult learning and in classroom teaching is going to be required. Again, an EMS service often chooses to bring in a training expert, but it certainly isn't essential if good internal people are available. Bear in mind, however, that outside experts sometimes have more credibility with employees than one of their peers.

Other considerations in the planning and designing of training require prior notification to those who'll be participating as well as allowing ample time for the preparation of all necessary training materials. There's nothing as embarrassing as having employees file into an ill-timed and poorly prepared training session.

■ Step 4. Prepare a budget or a cost-benefit analysis

In some cases, where training time is short, done on the job or performed as part of the expected duties of a regular employee (for example, a supervisor), little or no additional costs will be incurred.

In other situations, however, especially when outside trainers or programs are used, cost considerations are vital. In fact, the decision between hiring an outside instructor and using internal talent is often determined by budget considerations. Weighing the probable benefits against the projected cost (cost-benefit analysis) will usually result in an appropriate decision.

Delaying training, postponing it beyond a useful period or abandoning it altogether are obviously not helpful alternatives. If a problem needs fixing, and training appears able to fix it, it's not a good idea to put it off or drop it. All too often, EMS operators continue to muddle along, perpetuating the problem rather than approaching it head-on through appropriate training. Especially during bad times, training is sometimes seen as the least important priority, when in reality it should be the first.

■ Step 5. Gain management acceptance

While this may seem obvious, you'd be surprised how often operations' managers or others in middle management proceed with a training program for all the right reasons, only to have it mysteriously canceled at the last minute by an uninformed top manager. Top management should be kept informed. Active support is essential to the success of any training program. Sad are the stories of trainers who send graduates back to their jobs all steamed up about newly acquired methods of doing things, only to discover that their managers, determined to keep the old ways, have stymied the trainee's efforts. Managers can be great supporters and genuinely appreciative of training efforts *if* they've been previously informed of the expected advantages and have been given complete details of what their people are going to learn. In fact, if managers receive the training either along with or separate from the primary target training group, it can pay real benefits in terms of acceptance and reinforcement.

■ Step 6. Implement the program

In short *do* it! You've already decided on the program's objectives, the trainer, the materials, which learning activities you'll use and how it'll be evaluated. You've given yourself enough time for planning, notification and adequate preparation. Your management people support it, personally and financially. Go ahead! You're two-thirds of the way home.

■ Step 7. Evaluate results

Two thirds of the way? Right. Training doesn't stop when the lessons end. Now you're faced with the most important question of all. Did the training accomplish the intended results?

Presumably, you were careful to establish performance objectives that will make it easy to evaluate whether or not you got there ("telephone response time of five seconds or less"). Now all you have to do is measure. Are dispatchers actually answering the phones within five seconds? If they are, you're home free. If they're not, you're faced with the other one-third of the training job.

■ 8. Follow up

Successful companies in many fields know that follow-up is the most important phase of any operation. Were 100,000 new cars actually sold in the first month? Is brand X outselling brand Y? Is the telephone response time five seconds or less, 90 percent of the time? If not, why not? If dispatch telephone response time has risen to 10 seconds, something's obviously wrong. Either the training wasn't adequate or the dispatchers, for some reason, are reacting negatively to it. Perhaps the chief dispatcher wasn't properly informed and feels he has a better way, thus undermining your effort. It's your job to find out what's happened, and to take steps to assure it doesn't happen again. Most likely however, you'll have adequately gone through steps 1 through 6 and won't have these problems. But, they do happen. The point is to not quit but to instead avoid these pitfalls the next time by following up.

■ Step 9. Modify...and keep on keeping on

Since experience is the best teacher, there's no substitute for learning from your past successes *or* failures. Most of the time, modifications may only require a fine tuning—such as making sure the operation's manager is aboard the next time. Or you may only have to ensure that a spare projection bulb is on hand when you've scheduled a showing of the great film you have on a one-day $100 rental. Being able to make the difference between a great training experience and a mediocre or frustrating one is the mark of an effective trainer.

And now, back to steps 1, 2, and so on...funny thing about cycles. They repeat!

NOTES ON THE TRAINING PROCESS

To review some things to watch for.

Before starting your training program, be sure your needs are *training needs*, and don't reflect other problems.

Use *standards of job performance* to establish training performance objectives. These standards ideally begin with job descriptions. Compare actual performance with set standards in order to determine any discrepancies that training can reduce.

Carefully determine the *kind* of training needed. Are you trying to increase skills, change attitudes or what?

Select competent trainers who understand the learning process, and know how to use various training techniques.

THE ADULT LEARNING PROCESS

Just what does the adult-learning process mean? People learn when they're motivated to learn. This means that when folks are *rewarded* for learning, they'll want to learn more. The opposite, however, is also true—being punished for learning impedes the process. How can we reward learners? One way is to tell them how they're doing. When given *positive* feedback ("You're really doing great!") most learners will consider it a reward. When learners are able to master a task, then demonstrate it to others, the rewards from this accomplishment are great. When giving feedback, either positive or negative, remember that it's more meaningful when given immediately after the act rather than after time has elapsed and particulars forgotten.

Equally as important as motivating, is remembering that learning takes place through *doing*. Hearing or reading about it helps, but real learning happens through "hands-on" exercises.

The trainer, although in front of the class, is not the *only* teacher. Learners can teach and, conversely, teachers can learn! We can learn from one another. This is the value of conducting training as a group experience.

People learn in different ways and at different speeds. While it's true that most learn well by doing, some people learn well by just watching or listening. As trainers, we must recognize these differences and vary our teaching techniques accordingly. The use of slides, audio tapes, audio-visual tools, and so forth, will accommodate various learning styles.

People will often resist learning out of a fear of change or a dislike for the new job they're learning. It's important to recognize and minimize these barriers as much as possible. Time-management experts talk about a "swiss cheese"—approach. That is, taking a difficult assignment in small chunks and poking holes in it—hence swiss cheese. Most people accept learning best when it's delivered in bite-size pieces.

THE FOUR-STEP METHOD OF TRAINING

Most trainers agree that a four step method works best for most people.

1. Present the new information slowly, concisely and thoroughly.
2. Demonstrate the technique involved—show and tell.
3. Let the learner try it—mistakes and all.
4. Then correct where necessary, while gradually reducing your own role. Let the learner do it!

While these tips can't cover the entire field of training, they *are* intended to cover some basic training issues confronting EMS managers today. Remember one last axiom which serves most trainers well: *Above all else, and whatever the situation, BE YOURSELF.*

AVAILABLE RESOURCES

Most state EMS agencies have full-time training staffs available that will help EMS managers develop training programs. Also available are information packets with step-by-step guidelines for setting up various EMT and EMT-P programs. These state EMS agencies will sponsor instructor-training programs to help individuals improve their teaching skills and to encourage continuing education and in-service sessions.

Finally, available for loan is an extensive library of written and multi-media materials. This includes slides, videotape and film. For more information about these programs, write or call the training section of your state EMS agency (see Appendix F).

Dealing with Performance Problems and Discipline

Overview

If the most difficult person in your group were to blast into your office unannounced, throw the telephone through the window and accuse you of being stupid, you wouldn't have a problem deciding what to do with him. Unfortunately, it's never that easy. Most managers get in trouble by not handling the minor problems well. It's commonly believed that 10 to 15 percent of the subordinates cause 85 percent of the problems. They tend to cause problems four ways: (1) poor work quality, (2) low work quantity, (3) rule violations and (4) the inability to get along.

PURPOSE OF DISCIPLINE

The purpose of a disciplinary system is to create rules that are fair to everyone. Every manager has to be careful not to create a disciplinary work environment which solely enforces the rules or shows power and authority.

Generally speaking, EMS personnel want to work in a situation where performance expectations are reasonably strict. They don't enjoy working in an environment that isn't professional. They *like* to know the rules. They *want* to know where they stand. They *like* consistency. It's important for all to strive for success on a team where the coach is a bit demanding and where the rules are made to be obeyed.

The idea is to have an environment in which discipline is an educational process that demonstrates how the whole group benefits from compliance with the rules, even at the expense of personal freedom. Prehospital-care providers are usually quick to adhere to the rules once they see that others are involved and that they have a responsibility to their share of the rule-keeping.

It's crucial that all expectations are clearly defined in writing. When performance standards are stated clearly as part of the job description, or as a part of an overall performance objective system (for example, management by objective), there's no question when accepted standards of behavior deviate. Good organization and planning are vital to good discipline. A danger rests in fear of disciplinary action when punishment is used in such a way that people are afraid of losing their pay, job or prestige. They may become resentful, taking every opportunity to break the rules without getting caught. If the rules are too rigid, resentment builds in others and motivates them against you. If coaches, on the other hand, close their eyes to infractions, people will assume this indicates weakness and some will take advantage. Discipline breaks down and lack of respect for the rules results.

It's important that the rules remain and that the manager sees they're positively enforced. The manager who has good standards of discipline is likely to insist on high standards of work. Good communication skills are essential. It's important that complaints about rules are clarified immediately and that the boss is fair and doesn't play favorites. This is a part of the game all team members must play.

A manager's major responsibility is to keep his group's quality and quantity of work high. When an employee is under-performing, the manager must take action. The key is to handle the discussion with the employee in such a way as to motivate that person's team performance. The employee, however, must want to improve. If the improvement results because of threats, improvement will be short-lived with negative side effects. Such negative behavior may take form in complaints to fellow workers or subtle attempts to sabotage the effectiveness of the group.

KEY ELEMENTS FOR
IMPROVING PERFORMANCE

Have the employee focus on the problem. Many times the employee will avoid discussing the actual problem.

Ask for the employee's help in solving the problem. By doing this, you're indicating that you value the employee's ideas and experience. This enhances self-esteem.

If the employee introduces a useful solution to the problem, try to use his idea. Your use of the employee's good ideas will do much to enhance his self-esteem, which will eventually add to the overall team spirit.

It's important to handle problems early. When poor performance becomes apparent, and informal feedback hasn't produced the desired result, the supervisor should conduct a formal coaching or counseling session. This should be documented either as verbal or written counseling in case further discussions are required.

Coaching is the most effective technique for improving performance. Coaching steps are outlined in Figure 1.8. As a manager, preparing for a coaching session, consider Figure 1.9. It addresses what influences unsatisfactory performance.

Even though you've given the employee support and have had several discussions with him, you may not be able to resolve the problem situation. You then find yourself having to take disciplinary action in an attempt to resolve the situation. Of course, there are also instances in which you must take disciplinary action without having any previous discussions. When there are clear violations of the organization's policies or procedures, such as hazardous work infractions, theft or possession of illegal substances or firearms on

Figure 1.8   Steps of Coaching Technique

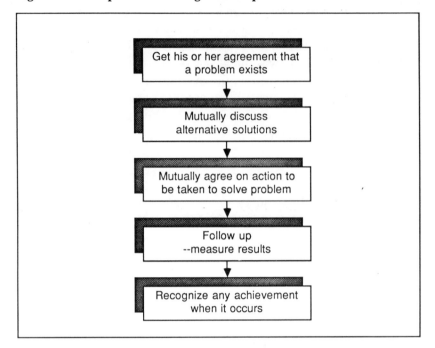

the premises, *immediate* disciplinary action becomes necessary.

The most effective disciplinary action requires several stages. The first action is generally the verbal warning or coaching session. If the verbal warning is ineffective, the next stage usually consists of a written warning. In further discussions, you may have to resort to more severe actions such as suspension, probation or termination.

Disciplinary suspensions have limited effectiveness in EMS situations. They hurt the organization in a number of ways. Often they increase the remaining staff members' workload, create overtime costs and are expensive if challenged through the legal process. Finally, the suspension's impact (which is supposed to cause the employee to think about his offending behavior) is often negated in short-staffed systems when the employee can earn lost wages with overtime in a few weeks. These are just a few reasons that should serve as strong motivators for supervisors and managers to intercede before issues get out of hand.

Disciplinary action is unpleasant for both the manager and the employee. Often the manager feels disappointed that the problem requires formal disciplinary action. At the same time, the employee

Figure 1.9   Coaching Decisions

What is influencing unsatisfactory performance?

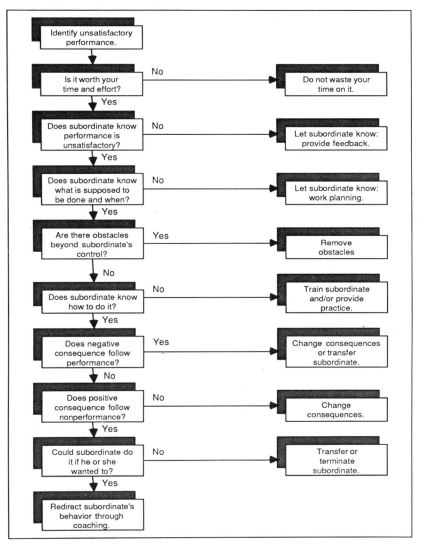

certainly doesn't like the disciplinary action taken and may feel it was uncalled for. The manager's objective is to have the employee understand the reason for the disciplinary action. Don't tell the employee that "it's company policy." Most employees won't accept this explanation. Explain your reason clearly: "When an employee violates the vehicle check-out procedure and begins a shift without the necessary ALS equipment, he is immediately given a 24-hour suspension to impress upon him the seriousness of the violation and its impact on patient care."

Don't be surprised if the employee reacts with hostility during the interaction. He may personally attack you as being "a poor supervisor." This type of hostility is understandable. The manager's or supervisor's objective is to use disciplinary action to encourage correct and appropriate behavior, while at the same time demonstrating that his support still exists.

Remember, disciplinary procedures should be progressive. Violations not handled in a progressive way should be stipulated in the employee handbook that the person is given when hired.

In any disciplinary action, the following should be used to achieve desired performance: *Describe* the situation, and review previous discussions. *Ask* the reasons for the situation. *Listen and respond* with empathy. *Indicate* what action you must take and why. Agree on a specific action and a follow-up date. And finally, *indicate* your confidence in the employee.

REASONS FOR DISCHARGE

Most reasons for dismissing ambulance employees fall into one of five categories: defective or negligent job performance, violation of organizational rules, fighting, challenging supervision or personal behavior.

Here's a quick run-down of common pitfalls encountered by ambulance services:

Defective job performance is hard to prove without clear standards of performance that are both measurable and documented, stating the employee had been advised in writing of inadequate performance.

Absenteeism, or just staying away from work, is cause for discipline. But if it results in firing, the service has the burden of proof that it's applied progressive discipline in a consistent way and has given ample warnings (such as suspension). Tardiness is also amenable to prompt and effective discipline.

Insubordination by an employee who challenges the supervisor, and threatens the power and authority of management, may result in termination. If the employee can prove that the insubordination was provoked, however, the dismissal may be overturned.

Off-duty conduct can *only* be a cause for discharge if it hurts the employer's reputation, business or interests. In fact, it's rarely a justifiable cause for termination.

Termination is a serious step for any manager to take. When you fire an individual and hire another to fill that position, you take the chance of exchanging one set of weaknesses for another. Although the person being terminated may be interfering with efficiency or causing discontent with other people on the job, any new person is going to have some weaknesses as well. It may be wise to first consider the advantages of the present employee.

The person in the job knows the company. He knows the policies, peculiarities, temperament and personality of the manager. Before you fire someone, ask yourself this: Have I done everything to help this person do the job right? A great deal of responsibility for his success rests on your shoulders.

When a manager hires a person, he's really saying, "I guarantee you can do this job. Furthermore, I guarantee that if you can't do it, I'll train and supervise you so that you can." Therefore, if the person isn't working out well, some questions the manager might ask himself are these: "Where have we failed?" "Have I lived up to my part of the deal?" "Is there anything more I can do to help this person?" "Would training, counseling or on-the-job coaching be advisable?" You should explore all the possibilities of working with a person before considering termination.

On the other hand, there are certain times when it's absolutely necessary to fire someone. If that person has developed bad work habits, if he's demonstrated immorality, dishonesty or incompetency, other people will be affected. People unwilling to change their behavior must go. One bad apple can cause others to spoil.

If an incompetent person stays around too long, people will say, "How long is the boss going to put up with him?" In order to get away from incompetency, good EMTs and paramedics may get restless and decide to leave. It's a reflection *on* management and a sign of weakness *in* management if inadequate or incompetent people are retained indefinitely.

At the beginning of the termination interview, the manager should explain to the person that he is being terminated, then review the facts, outline their past meetings and discuss how they have both tried to improve performance. Then the manager should point out the things that are below par in the employee's performance. A change must be made.

At this point, you may want to offer the person time off from work to look for another job, perhaps suggesting remaining vacation time. A sensitive manager can let the person tell others that he has decided to make the change. Regardless of the circumstances, when people are being fired, their self-esteem is low and they're vulnerable. They feel that they've failed and will be sensitive. Anything the manager can do to ease the departure will be helpful. Make sure the person's pay is arranged for a graceful and easy exit. Let the person save face if possible.

The important thing in firing someone is to do it so that everyone in the organization will say it was justified.

DEALING WITH TROUBLED EMPLOYEES

Alcoholism, drug abuse, emotional instability, illness and family crises are employee problems that frequently spill over into the prehospital-care organization. These problems, if not addressed, will affect a person's job performance. Personal crises involving marital, family, financial or legal problems are common in this high-stress work group.

An effective supervisor can help troubled employees in many ways, the most important of which is to be familiar with resources available that handle these issues. In relating to troubled employees, you should listen, be patient, discreet and reassuring. Employees should be encouraged to make an appointment to seek outside help. It's advisable to follow up to ensure that they're obtaining the necessary help and support. Generally, it's wise to listen honestly and sympathetically. Do what you can, within reason, to relieve his or her pressure. Refrain from giving specific advice. This is better left to professionals.

Even though you may want to be supportive, the manager can't compromise the service's mission. If employees aren't receptive to seeking help, make it clear that their continued employment will depend on their effective performance and that the problems affecting this performance must be solved.

C A S E   S T U D Y   # 2

The Troubled Employee

Ted Morrow looked down at the response-time reports facing him and, as before, the numbers beside Janet Thomas' name leaped up at him. For the fourth month in a row her out-of-chute time had increased—the time from unit dispatch to unit en route. In his years as an operations manager, he had seen this pattern all too often—an employee would be hired and perform well for a year or two and then, for no apparent reason, his or her performance would begin to slide. While the problem was always easy to spot, the cause commonly hid behind a hundred different reasons. It was his job to ferret out those reasons.

"Hi, Janet. Glad you could come by as soon as you did."

"Oh, it's no problem. I had a little bit of slack time anyway, so the timing's perfect."

"Janet, your supervisor just gave me your response-time reports for June. She noted that this report, in particular, is the fourth one in a row showing an increase in your out-of-chute time. You know that we think a lot of you as an employee, and I'd like to work with you to find out what's causing the problem."

"My supervisor mentioned that to me as well, and I really don't know what to say. It just seems that it's taking longer to get rolling on a call. It really bothers me, but I can't seem to do anything about it."

"Janet, I also reviewed your personnel records for the past year or so and learned something else. For the first eight months you were never late for work and were only absent once. During the past four or five months, though, you've been late 12 times and have used six days of sick leave—one day at a time. Is there a personal problem I need to know about?"

"No, not really. There've been some things that have come up around the house, but nothing serious."

"One other thing, Janet. And please understand that I'm discussing this because we care about you. It's been brought to my attention by others, and I've noticed it myself, that there seems to be a change in your attitude recently. You're not as cheerful and lively as you used to be—matter of fact, you seem somewhat short-tempered. You've also changed the way you dress. Now, I know this is all subjective and some of it might not even be any of my business, but it all points to a problem in your performance, and that *is* my business."

"I just don't know what to do. You're absolutely right. I feel so embarrassed to have everyone talking about me behind my back."

"Janet, it's only because they're concerned and want to help. What can we do to help you?"

"OK, Ted. You want to help? Try this. As you know, my husband, Jim, is the golf pro out at Greenbrier Country Club. Well, he's really popular, and the members love to get with him and talk shop in the lounge. I know this is normal for golf pros to do, and I didn't think much of it until I realized how much he was drinking around the house. When we were first married, Jim would usually have a six-pack around the house all the time but would rarely drink more than a can a day. Now he drinks a six-pack a day. He even has to have a beer to sleep at night. I think he's a full-blown alcoholic, but if I bring the subject up, it's a knock-down drag-out fight. That's number one.

"Number two is that about two months ago, while I was doing the laundry, I found a little bag of white powder in my daughter Shelley's jacket pocket. I asked her what it was. Eventually she admitted it was cocaine and that she had been using a little of it every now and again. She needs to go into a drug rehab program, but Jim says it's only a kid trying out stuff, that she's learned her lesson and to let the whole thing drop.

"So here I am, stuck right in the middle between an alcoholic and a drug user. It makes me so depressed, I just don't know which way to turn. Now, tell me how you're going to help."

Ted suddenly found himself in the middle of this personal, and yet not uncommon, situation. More and more often today, the complexities of everyday life invade the work environment. Managers, supervisors, foremen or personnel clerks must not only ensure that the work is being properly done, but must also play the role of part-time counselor and friend. Depending on company policy, Ted has a number of options. He can say, "Well, I understand you have problems, but you can't allow them to affect your daily work."—which would probably lead to her eventual dismissal.

A second alternative is the organization's employee-assistance program (EAP). Ted could continue to objectively measure Janet's performance and strongly encourage professional counseling for her and her family. He could also, throughout, assure her that things *can* improve.

The EAP conveys the organization's understanding that life embraces both personal time and time spent at work and that personal problems *directly* affect productivity and performance. Still, the EAP clearly separates the organization's role from an employee's personal life. It gets the manager, in this case Ted, out from in between and allows him to focus on the employee and the organization's mutual goals.

These are just two of the avenues open to a company with a nurturing and caring policy toward employees.

■ ■ ■

Performance Appraisal

"Even though it sometimes hurts, I appreciate it when a supervisor tells it like it is in my review."—AN EMPLOYEE

Overview

A manager once commented, "My EMTs don't want to be appraised. They prefer things go along as they are. They don't want to hear any bad news about how they're doing." Employees in this same service confided, however, that their appraisals weren't effective and that the manager simply used them to prove they didn't deserve a raise. Neither of these positions represent positive attitudes about performance appraisals. Independent research organizations have shown that employees regularly seek appraisals when supervisors and managers accurately identify both *accomplishments* and *shortcomings*.

REASONS WHY PERFORMANCE APPRAISALS ARE HELPFUL AND NECESSARY

Organizations that use performance appraisals effectively, regularly address the many important aspects of an employee's efforts and organizational expectations. Why are performance appraisals helpful?

Appraisals help people develop and grow. Feedback teaches employees how to take steps toward improvement.

Appraisals tell a company if its human resources are functioning. They answer questions for the company such as "What is our potential? How far have we gone? What expectations do we have for the future?"

Appraisals reward good performance and serve as an accurate measure for compensation.

Appraisals help correct deficiencies in poor performance. They provide checkpoints from which employees can review, reinforce or correct performance. They can also help revise performance targets.

Appraisals help assess various needs for further training, new-work assignments, rescheduling and so on.

Appraisals strengthen the relationship between the manager and each team member through a free and honest exchange. They help inform team members of the organization's expectations and allow those individuals to express their expectations back to management (a two-way process). If there's a real openness and involvement between manager and employee, an appraisal can motivate subordinates toward top performance.

REASONS WHY PERFORMANCE APPRAISALS DON'T WORK

It's been said that feedback is the breakfast of champions for managers. If so, why are performance appraisals so difficult? In many organizations, appraisals are nonexistent, random or useless. There are at least three reasons why.

Effective performance appraisals involve *confrontation*. They require facing up to disagreement and conflict. Many managers have trouble handling these types of confrontations. Others don't even try to manage them. They simply squelch any views different from their own. Many subordinates have trouble confronting the harsh facts in an appraisal. They prefer *not* to learn how competent or incompetent they are. The appraisal may make them feel threatened, embarrassed, angry, tense, resentful or hurt. In a defensive response they may argue, disagree, plead, shout, sneer, withdraw, sulk and belittle what the manager says. Performance appraisals can be heavy going. Many managers feel that they're just not up to this sort of thing.

Effective performance appraisals *take time*–lots of it. They can't be done in 15 to 20 minutes, once a year. Many managers aren't willing to invest the necessary time, so they don't do them, or they do quickie versions—slapdash appraisals that may do more harm than good.

Effective performance appraisals require *skills*–plenty of them. Many managers freely admit that they don't know how. And they're probably right. All too many appraisals are messed up by managers who know little or nothing about how they should be done.

HOW TO DEVELOP EFFECTIVE APPRAISALS

The basis for a performance appraisal is to compare results against agreed-upon goals. Goals are usually based on an employee's performance standards which have either become a part of that person's job description or have been established because of a performance-evaluation system such as MBO (management by objective). Each staff member should know what is expected of him, and those expectations should be measurable. Periodic appraisal interviews and regular performance updates are valuable in determining each employee's skill, motivation and level of satisfaction.

Performance appraisals should always be two-way. An employee should be given the chance to rate his job, work relationships and supervision. If there's openness and respect, a great deal of useful information can be gleaned from these sessions.

Good documentation of the individual's performance is necessary for a meaningful appraisal. Each session should be summarized and maintained in the employee's permanent record. Prior to each session, employees should update, in writing, their expectations and performance, and attach it to the formal evaluation that will become a part of their permanent record. Supervisors, physicians, nurse educators and the medical director should prepare written evaluations as well.

While the appraisal interview should be prescriptive, not remedial, employees should be encouraged to start with their feelings. Questions early in the interview such as "How have you seen your progress to date? What have you felt most pleased about? What are you most disappointed about in your own performance?" will help the employee relax and talk. By doing this, the employee may self-critique and provide feedback which will take pressure off the supervisor—he won't have to point out concerns and weaknesses. The employee's already doing it.

The interview must be performance oriented. Discussion of personalities, other individuals in the organization or patients should be minimal. Hidden agendas or other issues should be allowed to surface early. If dissension or distrust is apparent, it should be dealt with as it relates to the employee's performance.

The results of the appraisal shouldn't be a surprise to the employee if the service's supervisors have been involved throughout the review period. If there are surprises, it's a good indication that there are problems within the organization other than the *employee's* performance. At the conclusion of the interview, the employee should have a clear understanding of the supervisor's assessment, with an awareness of future expectations. In addition, there should be no remaining questions as to how performance was rated. If appropriate, there should also be a review of compensation as it relates to the appraisal.

Employees who receive high appraisals should get the highest pay increases. Management should consider them first for promotions when there are openings. Employees who receive low appraisals should receive coaching and assistance on how they can improve their performance. Everyone learns from effective performance appraisals. Employees learn what is expected, the organization gets better performance, and hopefully new avenues of communication for daily problem-solving are opened.

HOW TO MAKE PERFORMANCE APPRAISALS MORE USEFUL

Performance appraisals require absolute frankness. A supervisor who fails to report unsatisfactory performance blocks the paths of promising staff members. He's also judged on his inability to develop talent. In the same way, the supervisor who underrates his staff—sometimes to hoard talent—blocks the proper recognition and promotion of good employees. This failure to give due recognition frequently results in the employee's loss of initiative, if not resignation, and is costly to the overall operation of the service.

■ Preparing for the performance appraisal

Appraisals should be based on recorded accurate performance information. This ensures objectivity and fairness and provides the employee with specific and clear explanations. Every attempt must be made by the supervisor not to bias the rating with his own set of ideal personality traits or favoritism. The supervisor *must* remain objective. Previous appraisals shouldn't influence the current rating.

Ratings should reflect overall performance and not emphasize latest performance or an isolated dramatic incident which has already been corrected. This requires periodic notations of individual accomplishments. One performance's rating must not influence another's. For example, a poor rating for "cooperation" shouldn't influence the rating for "job knowledge." Each should be considered independently.

Grade level or length of service shouldn't affect the rating. Extensive experience or senior status doesn't necessarily mean good performance nor does brief experience mean poor performance.

Overall performance should be based on how well the employee has progressed in assignments since the last appraisal. In other words, the supervisor must approach his appraisal responsibility *not* to justify a salary recommendation, but to determine what level of achievement the employee has reached to merit a salary increase. Theoretically, a high rating should be followed by a high increase and vice versa. There are occasions, however, when this won't apply, such as when an employee is at or near the top of the salary range or when promotion isn't being considered.

■ Conducting the appraisal discussion

Supervisors are required to inform staff members of how well they've performed in their respective assignments. This is the appraisal program's payoff because it can further each employee's self-development. Scheduled employee discussions are, therefore, required with performance appraisals. However, don't forget that there are additional circumstances, such as transfers, promotions or corrective actions, when appraisals should be held as well.

Performance appraisals must be scheduled at regular intervals. Closer supervision of new staff members during their first year of employment will enable the supervisor to properly assess their development, attitudes, competencies and interests. A relatively inexperienced staff member may not understand all the elements of the job. As soon as possible, the supervisor should find out why this is so. It may be that a staff member gave an inadequate explanation of the specific duties involved because his orientation and training was too short. It's also possible that the new employee isn't suited by temperament or background to carry out his assignment. Any decision to transfer or terminate an employee should be reached during the first three months of employment.

The employee's potential within the service should be discussed during the appraisal. In certain situations, the supervisor may have to discuss the employee's potential in general terms. The reasons are twofold: to prevent a limited potential rating of a good employee from stifling the desire for improvement and to prevent employee dissatisfaction. If an employee receives an excellent or good rating, but his ambitions aren't fulfilled within a brief period of time, he may become dissatisfied. It's important the appraisal avoid both extremes, those of causing despair and of promises not possible in the short-range forecast.

There can be no doubt that a friendly and constructive performance appraisal can enlighten a staff member about his work and conduct. A person can't grow and develop in a job assignment if there's no yardstick against which to measure his performance. If commendation has been earned, this is a good time to give it. If there are certain weaknesses to overcome, this is a good time to tell him where improvement's needed and what can be done to improve his performance.

Some supervisors are reluctant to tell poorly rated employees how they stand. But consider how the supervisor would feel under similar circumstances. Not only do people prefer bad news over uncertainty, but staff members have the right to know where they stand and to receive corrective counseling before such drastic action as probation or termination is thrust upon them.

Although a properly conducted employee appraisal appears to be an informal and relaxed conversation, it's actually a carefully planned meeting for which the supervisor has fully outlined the areas to be discussed.

These additional guidelines will help a supervisor develop a positive appraisal climate.

Show that you have time for the interview and that you consider it important. Conduct it in total privacy.

Establish a constructive and helpful tone by emphasizing that the appraisal is being conducted for the employee's personal development and combined value to the service.

Be honest and straightforward in giving your evaluation, but allow "face saving" for the employee.

Be open-minded to opinions and information the employee may present, and be prepared to change your current evaluation in lieu of additional facts. Be alert to information which can help you learn more about the employee's short- and long-range aspirations.

Establish two-way communication. Allow the employee to get things off his or her chest without becoming defensive. Identify information presented and use it in such a way as to influence your objectives. Where possible, eliminate any general misconceptions the employee may have developed about individual assignments or service. Explain policy that is applicable. Remember, the supervisor is an important catalyst in uncovering staff dissatisfaction. And finally, keep in mind that faulty operational procedures can cause employee discontent. In such cases, it's the procedures—not the employee's behavior—that will need adjusting.

Conclude your discussion by telling the employee that you respect his feelings and, if rated well, that you're optimistic about his future. If he's been poorly rated, be frank about it, yet express that you know people can change. Explain that his current performance evaluation reflects his accomplishments within the past time period, but that it can be improved for future performance discussions.

During the discussion *do not* inform the staff member of any salary action you're recommending. Rather, indicate that any new salary information will be reported to him as soon as final approval has been given. The main reason for not divulging salary intent at this point is that a recommendation for a salary increase is often subject to change at higher levels.

If a salary recommendation is changed by higher levels (increased, reduced or disapproved), the decision should be fully explained to the supervisor so he can discuss it with his employee during follow-up meetings.

C A S E   S T U D Y   # 3

Performance Appraisal

Scene 1

As Mary Jo, the billing clerk, entered Linda Clark's offices she heard, "Well, it's performance-appraisal time. Guess we'll have to grit our teeth and get it over with."

The appraisal interview went down hill from there. "Well, I guess your attendance has been OK, but I know you've had some problems breaking in the new girl—can't give you a high mark on interpersonal relationships."

Breezing through the form, Linda seemed preoccupied. "I can only give you 15 minutes. Got several other people to do this with," Linda said, then took three telephone calls in succession. "It's not easy running this office," she remarked. As Linda's secretary loomed in the door, the office manager checked off the last item and handed the hastily completed form to Mary Jo. "Sign here," were her last words on the matter.

Without a chance to reply to any of Linda's assessments of her performance, Mary Jo left Linda's office with the feeling that it didn't much matter what she thought. "It's just another form, after all," she comforted herself.

Scene 2

Harry Green, the operations manager, was scheduled to meet with Bobby Breen, one of his field supervisors, later this afternoon. Harry dug through his files. There he found the data he was looking for— notes on three previous discussions he had had with Bobby, Bobby's attendance records, last year's performance appraisal, a letter documenting the incident in which Bobby had been involved with an irate patient. Harry felt well-prepared for Bobby's performance-appraisal meeting. He'd already completed his preliminary notes on Bobby's performance. He'd given Bobby a blank form to appraise his own performance. Now they'd sit down and compare notes. After that, having heard Bobby's own assessment, Harry would be able to provide a comprehensive appraisal. After all, he wanted to be as fair as possible and knew that Bobby would be as open with him as he planned to be with Bobby.

The interview went smoothly. Harry had set aside 45 minutes, and could make it an hour, if needed. He'd arranged to have his calls held and made it clear he wanted no interruptions.

At the conclusion of the interview, Bobby felt his views had been heard and that Harry had helped him see both the positive and negative sides of the way he handled his job. In fact, Bobby had rated himself lower on several categories than Harry had.

"This will really help me get ahead," Bobby thought. He was now planning to take some college courses, to attend a communications workshop, and to spend more time training his crew members. This was a result of the development plan he and Harry had worked out. "What's more," Bobby recalled, "Harry and I have gotten beyond some of our own communication barriers and can now be more open with each other. With the problems I've had, I can now see where it's important for me to make improvements. I never thought going through a performance appraisal would help me get along better with my boss and give me a clearer picture of where I can go in this company, but it did."

The first scenario is all too typical of performance appraisals within EMS. Rushed. Superficial. Of little help in developing more effective employees.

The second, much less familiar, goes to the heart of the objectives of good performance appraisals. Honest, based on objective data, of value to the appraiser and appraisee alike.

■   ■   ■

Part 1 dealt with the basics of personnel management and leadership, and introduced the importance of teamwork. The next step, critical to the success of every organization or team, is to understand the planning process.

2

Developing
The Game Plan

Planning

Overview

Simply defined, planning means deciding in advance what's to be done in the future. Through detailed planning, leaders attempt to achieve a consistent, coordinated and focused operational structure. Of course, plans alone don't bring about these results. But, without plans, activities will remain unfocused. Confusion and chaos then follow.

There are many excuses for not planning. Planning is mental work and for many ambulance managers, difficult. But there's no substitute for the hard thinking that planning demands. It's necessary to think before acting and to base action on facts rather than guesses. For this reason, planning is primary and precedes any other managerial function. Only after planning can a manager organize, staff, influence and control the team to accomplish the mission.

One way to look at planning is to see it as an organizational process with several steps. Beginning at the top of the organization, it's necessary to objectively define why you're in business—why the organization exists. What is your overall mission? Is it emergency medical service? Medical transportation? Prehospital care of the sick and injured?

(continued on next page)

(continued)

Having defined why you exist as an organization, some broad general goals can then be developed. But you need to be specific about how to reach your goals. That's where objectives with an accompanying plan come in. Spell out what needs to be done, by whom, when and how.

A common problem for prehospital-care organizations is a lack of systematic follow-through. This was confirmed recently when 20 services were informally and randomly surveyed to determine why their progress stalled and why they were unable to gain community and political support for a program. Of the 20 surveyed, only two indicated that they had written statements outlining their companies' goals and objectives that were updated quarterly. The other EMS managers gave dozens of reasons why they didn't. Some of the reasons included: "We save lives. I don't have the staff support for all that silly make-do paperwork." "We can't find enough hours in the day." Or, "We had planned to do it but something always came up." It should be no surprise that the two systems that had a written plan, well-known to all employees, that was used regularly, were the most successful.

There's no singular plan that will fit all EMS organizations. EMS organizations often use the same planning system of their parent organization or government unit. It doesn't matter what you call it, only that you do it. Each year it seems a new planning fad is on the horizon. What used to be called long-range planning is now strategic planning. Strategic planning is a significant part of the management process. Most of the advanced planning tools used today were developed from basic concepts found in management by objective. For that reason, we'll discuss it in more detail in the next section.

WHY PLAN?

The phone rings and the EMS unit's dispatched. Like a dog that barks on command, prehospital-care organizations often respond and

Figure 2.1   Planning Steps

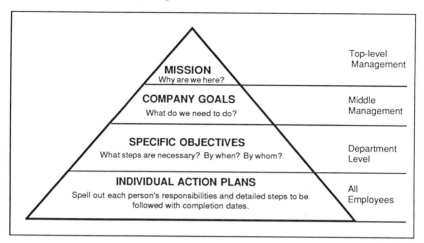

treat a patient's symptoms on demand. Many EMS managers promoted from within have likewise been conditioned by their field experiences to act in crisis. EMS leaders must do more than only respond to administrative symptoms. They must understand the disease process well enough to enable early detection and treatment before a crisis requires emergency intervention.

EMS leaders must become pro-active instead of re-active. They must direct the team's action before and during the "game" toward systematic goal completion rather than haphazardly reacting to isolated "plays" or incidents.

Management by Objective

Overview

Management by objective (MBO) has proven to be a valuable management tool in hundreds of health-care institutions over the past 25 years. Although the fancy term scares off many ambulance managers, MBO isn't difficult to understand or use. It provides a basis for planning and action in many aspects of the EMS system operation. It can be used effectively in human-resource management, financial management, information management, problem solving and planning.

It works because everyone in the organization becomes an active participant, a co-creator with managers, rather than just a spectator in determining the specific plans for the organization.

COMPONENTS OF MBO

MBO is the shared development of a plan with systematic checkpoints for follow-through. It's used by a manager much like a road map is used by EMTs when threading their way to an emergency scene. Similarly, MBO is the team's road map to the organization's successful completion of its mission.

The leader must understand the components of this management technique and be committed to its entirety. The components of an MBO system include *missions, goals, objectives, action plans, supporting policies and procedures* and *evaluation.*

The basic premise of this technique is that through self-control and clearly defined objectives, employees will become increasingly motivated. In this way, everyone in the service understands what needs to be accomplished, how it's to be accomplished, what their roles are and what type of performance is expected. Many ambulance services don't provide motivation and performance guidelines, or feedback, which helps increase productivity and satisfaction within the organization. The following actions discuss the specific components of the MBO system.

Figure 2.2 outlines the five steps to management by objective. The long-term goals are identified in light of the organization's mission. Specific objectives are created to meet these goals and a series of action

Figure 2.2   Five Steps To Management By Objective

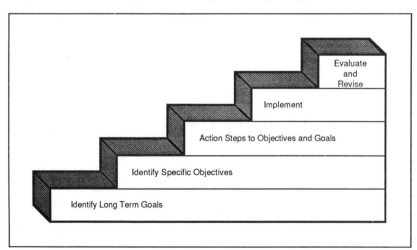

steps are prepared for members of the organization. After the system
is implemented, it must be evaluated and revised continuously.

■ Mission

The purpose of the organization's mission statement was
previously outlined. To review, it should answer the question "What
business are we in?"

■ Goals

Goals are the general tasks that an organization does to accomplish
its mission. An example of one of several goals within a year might
be to "increase the level of care from BLS to ALS."

■ Objectives

Objectives should be in writing. They describe what must be done
in order to achieve the goals. These objectives shouldn't be nebulous
pie-in-the-sky statements. Instead, they must be specific and
measurable. The objectives should say what's to be done, when it will
be done and who's going to do it. A limited number of objectives
should be established for any given period of time. A limit of five to
eight objectives is all most organizations can realistically accomplish
with success. Figure 2.3 describes specific criteria which should be
considered when writing performance objectives.

The process of establishing objectives should involve the
governing body as well as all managerial and supervisory personnel.
These individuals will assure the objectives fit the service's purpose
and plan. The manager is mainly responsible for this, but the people
responsible for supervising the activities should be included in
creating objectives and plans.

The objectives established must be S-M-A-R-T:

Specific
Measurable
Attainable
Relevant
Trackable

Specific. Effective action can't be taken on vague or confusing
objectives. If it is, there may be confusion and worse, apathy. For

Figure 2.3   Guidelines for Writing Performance Objectives

1. It starts with the word "to", followed by an action verb.

2. It specifies a single key result to be accomplished.

3. It specifies a target date for its accomplishment.

4. It specifies maximum cost factors.

5. It is as specific and quantitative (and hence measurable and verifiable) as possible.

6. It specifies only the "what" and "when"; it avoids venturing into the "why" and "how".

7. It relates directly to the accountable manager's roles and missions and to higher-level roles, missions, and objectives.

8. It is readily understandable by those who will be contributing to its accomplishment.

9. It is realistic and attainable, but still represents a significant challenge.

10. It provides the desired payoff on the required investment in time and resources.

11. It is consistent with the resources available or anticipated.

12. It avoids or minimizes dual accountability for achievement when joint effort is required.

13. It is consistent with basic company and organizational policies and practices.

14. It is willingly agreed to by both superior and subordinate, without undue pressure or coercion.

15. It is recorded in writing, with a copy kept and periodically referred to by both superior and subordinate.

16. It is communicated not only in writing, but also in face-to-face discussions between the accountable manager and those subordinates who will be contributing to its attainment.

example, the objective for an unenlightened service might read: "The service shall be more responsive to patients." A vague statement, to be sure. No one can act on this objective. A more specific and more readily implemented statement might be, "The service shall reduce response times on priority-one (life-threatening) calls."

Measurable. Even though the latter statement is more specific, how can a manager determine if it's been carried out? Exactly what are the subordinates being held accountable for, and how is performance going to be measured? What does a good job look like? Instead, the objective should read, "Reduce the response times on priority-one calls. Our goal by September 1, 1988, is to expect 90 percent to have response times of less than eight minutes."

Attainable. The next step in evaluating the objective is to determine whether the goal is attainable. Past history, available resources and commitment are used to determine if a goal is realistic. Using the above example, if the service currently has response time of less than eight minutes for 40 percent of the time, 90 percent compliance might not be a realistic expectation, unless significant financial and human resources are directed toward its attainment. Even attainable objectives, however, should include some stretch. They should challenge the organization and be difficult enough to increase commitment and creativity.

Relevant. Is the objective relevant? It's commonly considered that about 80 percent of the performance desired from workers is derived from 20 percent of their activity. Is the objective important enough to devote the time and resources necessary for its accomplishment? Are there more important objectives to be emphasized? More importantly, does the objective support and enhance the organization's mission? The mission statement of the organization is "to provide the region with the highest quality prehospital medical care and transportation with the resources available." In this example, there is a direct relationship between the quality of care and the response-time objective. Therefore, this would probably be an appropriate and relevant objective for the organization.

Trackable. The final component of an effective objective is its ability to be monitored. Is it trackable? Records must be kept to follow the person's performance in attaining the objective. If there is no record system, start one! That way the manager can frequently measure performance. This will provide a method to determine the success of the organization toward the accomplishment of objectives. It will also help provide feedback to subordinates on how well their work is supporting or not supporting goal attainment.

After performance objectives are created and accepted, the team must determine which of the objectives are most important. This enables the service's resources to be directed in the most meaningful direction.

The diagram in Figure 2.4 demonstrates the relationships among the MBO steps in enhancing the mission of the organization. The similarities between Figure 2.4 and Figure 2.1 are evident.

■ Action Plans

Action plans, or steps, are those individual tasks that must be completed to reach the objective. Individual employees are usually

Figure 2.4   Example of MBO in Action

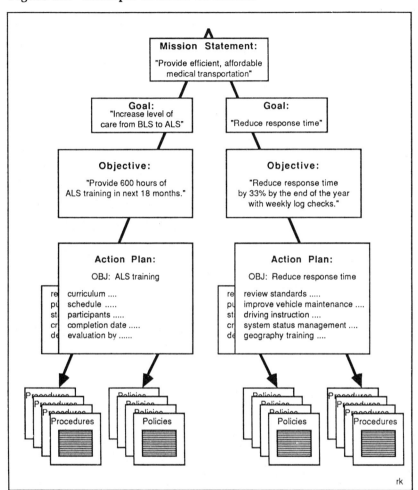

involved in the completion of these steps. They should understand their role in the completion of the task and know in very specific terms what's expected of them. They should also be aware of how each step helps satisfy the objective, why the objective was created and how it fits into the organization's overall mission.

■ Supporting Policies and Procedures

These are the meat of the plan. When policies and procedures are written or are modified to support the plan, it demonstrates the leadership team's commitment to the plan. It also emphasizes that they're being created or modified to prepare the organization for the implementation of the plan.

■ Evaluation

The major reason for monitoring ongoing performance is to enable the manager to provide feedback to subordinates and leaders. Feedback from someone who has the big picture helps keep employees focused on the objective. The monitoring phase also demonstrates that the leader is informed and aware of the necessary steps. Continuous monitoring of performance permits the team to stay on target by making interim decisions and revisions during the target period. Both favorable and unfavorable trends can be observed during monitoring. This allows the organization to respond to changes in service patterns, the economy or other outside influences.

It's important that all personnel involved in planning be regularly updated on how well they're doing regarding the achievement of goals. Many people are motivated by achievement, and for them feedback can act as a catalyst for further achievement. For those less motivated, feedback may provide the encouragement necessary to increase their performance. Everyone in the organization needs to be aware of his individual performance as well as the organization's effectiveness in meeting its targets. One ambulance service found it effective to create a wall-size mural in their conference room to monitor team members and keep them abreast of their progress.

The day-to-day operational monitoring of the work directed toward reaching the objectives provides a guide to required action during the target period. Individuals must know how well or how poorly they're performing. The team must be able to identify, as soon as possible, when plans are not working. Otherwise, corrective action can't be taken to keep the goals realistic. In the absence of timely and meaningful feedback, the leader runs a strong chance of losing control of the operation and having the objectives and plans become obsolete.

Figure 2.5 shows how feedback can make the organization more responsive to variances—a divergence from expected targets. As you can see, action toward a deviation can be taken faster and more efficiently when proper monitoring mechanisms are in effect and feedback processes are decentralized. Through this process, the leader and individual employees become aware of variances sooner so they can get the plan back on track.

Figure 2.5   Traditional Versus Decentralized Feedback

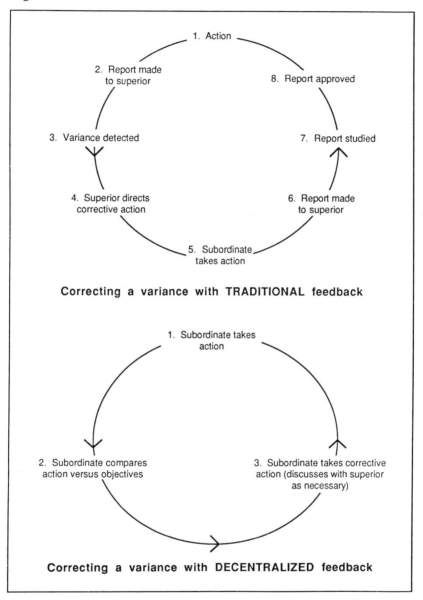

Correcting a variance with **TRADITIONAL** feedback

Correcting a variance with **DECENTRALIZED** feedback

MBO requires that meaningful feedback be tailored to the objective of each person involved in planning. Following is a five-step plan to help tailor your feedback to each employee's needs:

1. State the objective.

2. Define how you will monitor performance.
3. Discuss how often you'll provide feedback. This will depend on how often the employee is in a position to take remedial action.
4. Determine who should get copies of the report.
5. Describe the report's form. The simpler the better.

This plan provides effective feedback to ensure people are aware of their performance toward the goal. In this way, MBO provides accountability at every level of the organization and can become an integral part of its performance-appraisal system. MBO is a more personal orientation to an appraisal because individual, and often personal, objectives can be set in addition to organizational objectives.

HOW DO WE KNOW IT WAS DONE WELL?

Results. That's how. In short, the organization must perform or everyone in it will know why. In this way, the organization performs against measurable standards that assure competence from top to bottom.

In summary, MBO can be a powerful tool to accomplish multiple managerial functions within an EMS service. This includes planning, organizing, influencing and controlling the organization. A brief overview of the process has been presented here. A number of articles and textbooks have been written on this subject. Further study should be considered before implementing an MBO system for your ambulance organization.

Problem Solving— A Workable Model for EMS

Overview

Most EMS managers have had the experience of having three crises erupt while having their first cup of coffee. A "good crisis" to many managers is like a "good trauma call" to paramedics. Unfortunately, managers don't always make the best decisions when operating in a crisis or when otherwise under pressure. The effective manager must learn to handle pressure so that reasonable solutions can be developed—solutions the entire team can live with.

Every manager is involved in problem solving, whether policy, organizational, technical or interpersonal. Many times, situations don't represent new problems, just recurring ones. To avoid breakdowns in problem solving, pay careful attention to methodology.

STEPS IN PROBLEM SOLVING

The following steps will help resolve any problem. Omitting any one of these steps, regardless of how simple or complex it may seem, will leave the solution to chance rather than a planned resolution.

Define the problem. Field personnel usually treat symptoms, not the underlying disease. Likewise, ambulance managers often describe issues. The exact nature of the underlying problem must be clear to everyone involved in its solution. To locate the exact conflict, ask yourself these questions. Who's involved in the conflict? What specific data suggests that there *is* a problem? What kind of a problem is it—is it one of understanding, attitude or competence? What does the problem seem to demand from the manager?

Involve every person. Every person involved in the problem must feel an important part of the solution. If he doesn't feel involved in the decisions, he won't care what the outcome is. To check involvement, the manager should ask, How willing are those involved to accept the consequences of their proposed solution? How well represented are those with expertise in this area? How well represented are those who are affected by the decisions?

Clarify. Focus on the basic problem. Other issues should only be considered while focusing on the main issue. The primary problem may even change during this stage. If such is the case, everyone involved must be aware of the changes. To limit the problem, ask, What is the central issue? What is at stake? What is the cause?

Review. Periodically evaluate any progress by asking these questions. How much agreement is there on the problem? Have all involved felt free to express themselves? Has the actual problem been described or just its symptoms?

Solve. Do some brainstorming. Test all possible solutions without elaborating or evaluating. Premature criticism may stop the creative flow of ideas. Encourage what may seem like impossible ideas—they may not be so farfetched. When the list is completed, see if any of the suggestions can be combined. Here are two helpful questions to ask. What would be the best outcome? If there were unlimited resources available, what could be done with the problem?

Experiment. Each proposed solution should be pretested using standard criteria to assess its workability and to narrow its choices. Even then, since some solutions can't be thoroughly tested, it may be necessary to act without certainty. What help can be expected and from whom? What has been the experience of others? What should be modified and how?

Plan. Putting a solution into effect requires careful planning in terms of specific individual responsibilities. No one can adequately carry out a plan without being fully informed of the manager's expectations. Planning for action includes planning for evaluation. What's to be done? Who is to do it? When is it to happen? How is it to be evaluated?

Act. No problem is solved unless someone does something about it. A plan needs to be implemented by the assigned person and monitored at each stage to compare the results with the original plan. Questions on taking action you might ask yourself are, How can the situation change? When will the action take place?

Evaluate. A review of the action taken may show that the original problem was solved. Or a review may help avoid repeating mistakes. More typically, the action taken uncovers new problems, and the process begins again. Few problems are completely solved. Helpful questions at this stage are What evidence is there of permanent improvement? How adequate have the problem-solving procedures been? What new problems have been identified?

These steps may at times seem overly complex and tedious. However, once the ambulance manager internalizes the process, it becomes easier. EMTs and paramedics are taught to use a standard format in communicating medical information to a physician at the base hospital to avoid omitting important facts. Likewise, managers who follow this protocol for problem-solving will avoid missing vital information that may affect the outcome. Remember, there are no real problems—only opportunities!

C A S E   S T U D Y   # 4

Problem Solving

There's a serious backlog in billing. Susie, the office manager, has asked for help. Operations personnel and other office personnel with time available have refused to help. "It's not my job," they say. The fact is that a peak period, with an unusually high volume of runs, has just passed and now there appears to be some slack. Therefore, Susie feels that it's appropriate to ask others to help.

What's the real problem? Let's define it clearly.

STEP 1: Definition of the problem

Q. Who's involved? What suggests there *is* a problem?
A. Conflict between office and field personnel.

Q. What kind of problem is it?
A. One of understanding (the office needs help) and of attitude ("I'm an EMT. Don't bother me with billing problems.").

Q. What does the problem demand from the manager?
A. The manager needs to encourage teamwork from his staff for the benefit of the service.

Comment: Although the problem does involve billing, the real problem is lack of teamwork among employees.

STEP 2: Involvement

Q. How willing is the staff to face problems and accept the consequences of a solution?
A. There's a real need to develop greater willingness.

Q. How well represented are those with expertise?
A. Susie is prepared to take the lead.

Q. How well represented are those who will be affected?
A. All will be affected if billing isn't done. This message and its consequences need to be communicated.

STEP 3: Clarification

Q. What's the central issue?
A. A need for greater teamwork.

Q. What's at stake?
A. The profitability of the service as well as its ability to maintain financial integrity, which includes payment to employees.

Q. What's the cause?
A. This is hard to define. The next step will help.

STEP 4: Review

Let's say at this point that Susie has already attempted to communicate some of these issues to staff, but has failed to gain cooperation.

Q. How much agreement is there on the problem?
A. Very little.

Q. Have all felt free to express themselves?
A. Apparently, although we might question the degree to which full communication took place.

Q. Has the actual problem been described or just the symptoms?
A. It appears that only the symptoms have been addressed.

STEP 5: Solution

Now the manager is likely to want to brainstorm some possible solutions with key people, certainly including Susie. Some possible ideas could include:
> —Order certain staff to work with Susie on billing.
> —Issue a directive censuring the staff for their lack of team spirit.
> —Hold a meeting to communicate the real issues, and seek volunteers.

After discussing the list of alternative solutions, the manager and his key staff may see the first two suggestions as unworkable, or at least likely to cause additional conflict, and settle on the third as the most desirable.

Q. What help can be expected? From whom?

A. With the problem clearly communicated, there should be a high level of cooperation.

Q. What has been the experience of others?

A. The service in a neighboring county has always worked in this manner, so have many other organizations we know of.

STEP 6: Plan

Q. What's to be done?

A. A staff meeting will be called.

Q. Who is to do it?

A. The general manager.

Q. When?

A. Tomorrow morning at 8:30

Q. How is it to be evaluated?

A. By the degree of support shown.

STEP 7: Action

Do it! Simple enough! But, bear in mind that this could be seen as a sensitive issue and may set a precedent for the organization. Care needs to be taken to reinforce the team concept on an ongoing basis, and to provide some recognition for those who step forward to assist.

STEP 8: Evaluation

How did it work? In this case, there is the likelihood for improved teamwork throughout the organization. Yet, some new problems may have been identified. These could involve some individuals not feeling "on board" and the issue of ongoing activities, to reinforce the new teamwork concept.

■ ■ ■

Manager's Checklists

Overview

The activities of the EMS manager are discussed throughout this book. Over and over, routine control and monitoring are emphasized. It's impossible to tell how well a manager is doing, however, unless there are standards and ways to measure activity.

The management skills outlined earlier are tools to achieve results. The true measure of the manager's effectiveness is the results achieved by the total team. For example, how well is the service performing the mission of the organization? The manager must continually monitor this performance in an objective, unemotional way. Figure 2.6 is a manager's list of activities and information which he must routinely review. This list is by no means complete, but should serve as a guide upon which a manager can build.

Figure 2.6 Manager's Checklist

DAILY	WEEKLY	SEMI-MONTHLY	MONTHLY
Review: Status of vehicles Previous day's revenues, runs, charges, & deposit News reports Incident reports Complaints Staffing	Review: Personnel scheduling Responses & response times Unit hours scheduled Unit hours consumed Straight-time equivalent (STE) hours scheduled STE consumed Hours lost due to injury, illness, or vacation Number of times call-in was required and for how long	Review: Bank balances Payroll Overtime Prepare: Accounts payable	Review: Statistical indicators Balance/P & L statements Run analysis Time analysis Trade journals General ledger Patient reviews Inventory Prepare: Agenda for Board Report for Board Comparison of budget to actual

QUARTERLY	SEMI-ANNUALLY	ANNUALLY
Review: Existing plans and objectives Prepare: New plans for objectives For patient audits	Review: Accomplishment of employee goals Perform: Performance appraisals Employee social activity/awards/recognition	Review: Personnel policies Medical protocols Corporate objectives Service & vehicle licensing Taxes Financial audit Investments Vehicle & equipment needs Insurance policies Prepare: Annual goals and objectives Budget Year end reports

This is only a partial listing of the manager's tasks. The importance of this guide is to emphasize the necessity of planning and scheduling activities.

Figure 2.7   Sample of Manager's Weekly Operations Summary

WEEKLY OPERATIONS SUMMARY
for
CRISS CROSS AMBULANCE DISTRICT

From: _____ hrs./on _____ - _____ 198_   To: _____ hrs./on _____ - _____ 198_

STATISTICAL INFORMATION:

	TOTAL	EMERG	NON-EMERG	LONG DIST.	OTHER	% of TOTAL
Responses						
Transports						
Canceled--prior to arrival						
Mutual aid						
Not transported						

Emergency response times over: 10 minutes _____
15 minutes _____
20 minutes _____
30 minutes _____

UNIT HOURS:

Unit hours scheduled _____
Unit hours consumed _____
STE/payroll hours
scheduled   _____
STE/payroll hours
consumed   _____

PERSONNEL:

Lost Hours:
_____ Vacation
_____ Illness
_____ Injury

Number of times call-in
required: _____

MEASURING YOUR SERVICE

Much of the information reviewed by the manager must be provided by reports. Figure 2.7 is an example of a weekly report for the manager. This details current activity and the status of the nuts-and-bolts operation of the service. An effective manager is well informed and must know what's going on at all levels of the organization. The manager remains aware by evaluating and measuring the performance of the system. This is done by adhering to established reporting methods as well as by verifying these reports through observation. Talking with team members, officials and patients is also important.

The reporting system can be divided into various areas, which collectively give a picture of the entire service. These areas include the following:

Operations:
   Ambulance runs: locations, destinations, types, response times
      and times of calls.
   Patient assessment and diagnosis
   Personnel-production activity: "out of chute," "droptimes,"
      absenteeism, licensure, turnover, and so on.
Financial:
   Charges and cash receipts
   Accounts receivable
   General-ledger accounting
   Balance sheets, operating statements
   Statistical indicators

Some reports may have information for both financial and operational areas. Some may be specifically designed to measure one particular activity. An entire book could be written about managerial reporting systems. Only a few of the important items are described as examples.

The section dealing with System-Status Management in Part 4 (page 214) details the importance of time-of-day and location reporting, and how this information can be put to use. The length of calls and destinations are also important data.

Many services must meet strict response-time criteria for various calls. Traditionally, the measurement was based on average-response times. This means of measurement is deceptive. A service can have an adequate average response time and still not reach a great proportion of its patients within an acceptable time frame. There is a better way to measure response times called Response-Time Performance Percentages (RTPP). This measures what percentage of the time each type of call is answered within a specified desired maximum limit. For example, the service is required to respond to 90 percent of all priority-one calls within eight minutes or the service is to respond to all priority-two calls within 10 minutes. This gives a better idea of the service's performance. Some services may need to calculate these response-time performance percentages for various areas served.

Assessment reports simply give the manager a "mix" of the type of patients being transported based on specific injuries or types of illness.

Reports designed to make sure all field personnel are current for licensure and training are helpful. It's necessary to keep track of sick time, vacation time and the number of personnel on duty during various periods. It's also possible to develop a reporting system which provides information on response times, percentage of no-hauls, amount of supply use and other information for specific crew members or ambulance units.

Figure 2.8   Sample Statistical-Indicators Report

CRISS CROSS AMBULANCE DISTRICT
Statistical Indicators

	April Actual	April Budget	Year to Date Actual	Year to Date Budget
Total Calls	313	348	1,360	1,393
Average Calls Per Day	10.43	11.61	11.33	11.61
Total Miles Traveled	6,940	6,380	24,009	25,518
Vehicle Cost Per Mile of Operation	0.63	0.72	0.73	0.72
Personnel Cost Per Patient	128.76	130.27	119.13	130.27
Total Operations Cost Per Patient	214.20	192.53	184.02	192.53
Gross Revenue Per Patient	222.80	194.90	204.30	194.90
Total Personnel Cost Per Day	1,034.40	1,202.38	1,047.33	1,202.38
Total Operations Cost Per Day	1,720.73	1,777.04	1,617.86	1,777.04
Average Daily Collections	1,142.30	1,169.31	1,071.48	1,169.31
Average Daily Revenues	1,789.83	1,798.94	1,796.16	1,798.94
Average Days in Accounts Receivable	90.8		90.5	
Total Unit-hours	1,608	1,680	6,553	6,720
Labor Cost Per Unit-hour	16.33	18.67	16.21	18.67
Ratio of Patient Transports / Unit-hour	.15	.16	.16	.16
Collection Rate (%)	63.8%	65.0%	59.7%	65.0%

Figure 2.9   Unit-Hour Analysis

The following steps will enable you to calculate the number of unit hours your service provides each week. It will also calculate the utilization (transports per unit hour). The cost of providing a single unit-hour is also determined as the final step. Use the same one-month period for performing all of the calculations below.

1. Calculate the number of hours all ambulances are staffed and on duty for each week. (For example one ambulance on duty 24 hrs. a day, seven days a week will equate to 168 unit hours. 24 hrs. X 7 days = 168 unit hours. An ambulance staffed 8 hours, 5 days per week would provide 40 unit hours. 8 hrs. X 5 days = 40 unit hours.) Total all ambulance hours provided by your service.

   Total unit hours for one week = (A.) _____ *unit hours.*

2. Determine the average number of transports per week. Take the average number of transports (not requests) for the month and divide by the number of weeks (This will not be an even number--for example a month with 31 days will have 4 3/7 weeks).

   Average transports per week = (B.) _____ *transports per week.*

3. To calculate the unit hour utilization, divide the number of transport per week (B.) by the number of unit hours (A.).

   Unit hour utilization = (B.) ÷ (A.) = _____ *transports per unit-hour.*

4. Determine the expenses per week, by dividing the total expenses for the month by the number of weeks. The number of weeks should be identical to the number in "2". (Total expenses for the month ÷ number of weeks.)

   Total expenses for a week = (C.) $ _____ *per week.*

5. This allows the calculation of the total service cost per unit hour. To determine this divide the total expenses for one week by the number of unit hours per week. (Total expenses per week (C.) ÷ (A.) Total unit hours.)

   Cost per unit hour = (C.) ÷ (A.) = $ _____ *per unit hour.*

All services have reports devoted to monitoring financial information. One financial and operation report that deserves special attention is the Statistical Indicators Report which can give the manager current information on the service's performance. This monthly report demonstrates a variety of trends that indicate production and financial activity. Figure 2.8 shows information one service found useful in its Statistical Indicators Report. Most of the information is self-explanatory. An important concept to measure service is the unit-hour concept. Figure 2.9 is a worksheet to help managers determine unit hours. Unit hours are also discussed in the section on scheduling entitled System Accountability Through Improved Personnel Scheduling (page 201).

A manager can't monitor or control without comprehensive reports. Well-run professional services realize the value of this practice.

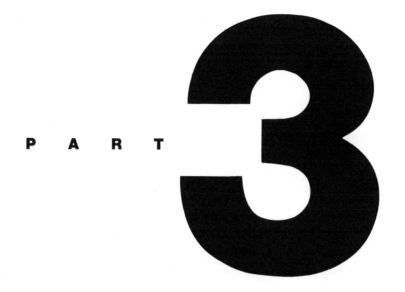

P A R T **3**

The Buck
Starts Here

Money Matters

Overview

You may be thinking "The Buck Starts Here" is a foolish title for this part. It was chosen because we wanted a *not-too-subtle* reminder that it all starts with the patient and service to that patient. Without patients, ambulance services would have no reason to exist. Think about it. This thought is crucial to *every* prehospital-care and medical-transportation provider in America. There's no one "right" way to finance an ambulance service. It's important, however, that managers understand the responsibility inherent in ambulance service work. To do this they must act thoughtfully regarding financial matters in order to maximize the benefit to patients.

Financial planning and control are perhaps the most difficult skills for EMS managers to master. Like new pilots learning to anticipate and control an airplane's movements, they must master these skills or their "plane" will crash. Whose responsibility is it to see that a system is financially stable? The manager must accept responsibility as "the pilot." Many managers list the political climate, high employee wages, low tax subsidies, poor collections and a variety of other excuses for their service not being financially successful.

(continued)

To do so is like saying the airplane passengers are responsible for controlling the aircraft. Think of it this way, how many commercial airline crashes few years were caused by *passenger error?*

And now for the answers to some commonly asked money-matter questions. The questions are easy—the answers are tough!

QUESTIONS AND ANSWERS

Where does the money come from? Most services get their support from tax subsidies, patient revenues, service charges or subscriptions. Any one or a combination of these methods can be used to finance the service. In addition, many volunteer organizations are supported by donations, fund-raising activities and bequests.

How does the service get the money? The ways of obtaining these revenues are as varied as the number of services themselves. Tax-supported services usually participate in an annual budgetary process. This leaves the service at the mercy of the political process and may require the manager to spend an inordinate amount of time in turf battles. In addition, many public services, and every proprietary service, use a billing and collection process that obtains revenue directly from the patient or from a third-party payer. Most EMS managers get hung up with the term third-party payer. To many, it's an impenetrable wall behind which lurk sinister people who prevent the service from meeting its goals. Not so. They're actually nice people who simply don't want to give up any more of *their* money than they have to. If you don't ask, or don't know what to ask in order to shake the dollars loose, don't expect them to deliver a money tree for your service.

The most important issue regarding where the money comes from is the relationship among subsidies, charges and reimbursement. Services that receive high subsidies usually have low charges or rates. Since the ominous third-party payers only pay a portion of this amount, the service's rate of reimbursement also remains low. It's a vicious cycle that doesn't benefit the patient, the service or the community. The real winners are the insurance companies. The insurance companies don't have to pay for the full cost of the service. Instead, they pay the artificial lower cost which is supplemented by the taxpayers.

Protection from high rates has been an ongoing justification for the existence of many poorly managed services that charge little or nothing. Low rates and poor reimbursements are the explanations given by these same services as to why their service is poor.

Local elected officials have begun to realize that a part of every dollar of local EMS tax subsidy is really a gift to the federal government and private insurance carriers. These same local officials are investing their subsidies at a time when the feds are drastically cutting support to local communities by wiping out revenue sharing. At the same time insurance companies are raising their rates.

Public services are realizing that charging rates lower than the direct cost of providing the service undermines the medical-care profile. This creates future financial nightmares and threatens all surrounding services, both public and private.

How does a manager plan for where the money goes? Detailed budgeting is the answer. A coach who fails to plan a strategy for the game doesn't win many games. The same is true with budgeting for ambulance services. The manager must anticipate what the costs will be in order to provide adequate service during that period. There are two rules for budgeting.

1. Every expense can be anticipated and budgeted.
2. If rule number one doesn't work, there should be a contingency plan to cover it.

How does one know "how it's going—financially?" The EMS manager must become proficient at reading financial statements, interpreting their contents, spotting unfavorable financial trends and knowing what to do about them. It's been estimated that over 70 percent of the ambulance services have inadequate financial monitoring systems. Financial statements can be likened to your team's scoreboard. If the coach reads the scoreboard and sees that you're behind early enough in the game, corrective action can be taken to pull it off. However, if you don't look at the scoreboard until the end of the game... well, you know what happens.

How can the money be protected from dishonest individuals? A familiar phrase is emblazoned on U.S. coins: "In God we trust." That's OK, but the advice here is to suspect all others. The easiest way to avoid going to jail, or wanting to place one of your co-workers there, is to develop a system of procedural checks and balances that discourages *anyone* from dipping into the till. This should include, at a minimum, an annual independent review of the organization's financial records.

How does one know that the funds are being spent wisely? Again, the answer is to instill procedures that "idiot-proof" the service from a person's poor judgment and extravagance. This can be done through appropriate purchasing, inventory and accounting procedures.

"Are we having fun yet?" Don't quit now! The gory details are yet to come. Seriously, each of the items touched on are covered in greater detail in the following sections. It's hard reading, which is why you've been exposed to the short course first.

Budgeting

Overview

The financial future of any emergency-medical or patient-transport organization is established through budgeting. A budget can be defined as *a planning and control system.* It's a financial action plan which the organization intends to follow for a specified period of time. It's not a one-time computation of numbers to satisfy obligations, but rather a continuous process throughout the budget period, generally one year. A budget shouldn't be created and then stuffed in a drawer until next year. It should be referred to regularly and compared with what is happening financially in the organization.

There are four main objectives to EMS budgeting. A budget provides, in measurable terms, a *written* expression of objectives, policies and plans of the service. It provides a basis for evaluating financial performance in accordance with the plan. A budget provides a useful tool for cost control (tool only!). A budget helps to create financial awareness *throughout* the organization.

Budgeting gives the ambulance manager a benchmark for monitoring the flow of dollars in and out of the organization.

(continued on next page)

(continued)

It forces the governing board, management and staff to write a plan for handling funds. It also requires the organization to relate this plan to its overall goals and objective. The budget provides a means for evaluating financial performance. It measures what was predicted against the stark reality of what actually occurred. It can be used to identify areas which are costing too much or where mistakes were made in the forecast of events. By involving the entire organization in budgeting and the company's budget goals, everyone is better informed about the operation and direction of the service.

Budgeting establishes realistic goals and objectives by requiring the service to measure expenditures against revenues. It requires that all activities be coordinated into the overall plan. It provides a standard against which the actual results can be measured, and a basis for effective cost control, planning and allocation of people and funds.

Budgeting requires that the service determine the financial feasibility of programs before including them in the organizational plan. This ensures that the new programs are realistic and attainable and that the organization has the financial resources to accomplish them. Budgeting also requires activity coordination. Finally, it provides a tool with which to measure the performance of the different activities.

There are three things the manager must have before preparing a budget. He must have a *commitment* from the governing body and the administration to follow both the plan and the budget. The manager, himself, or someone he appoints, must *monitor* the budget on a regular basis, and that person must have the authority *to act* if unfavorable variances from the budget are observed.

It's important to remember that the budget isn't just a list of numbers, but a statement of objectives and specific plans for reaching organizational goals. An effective budget is well documented and consists of five parts:

1. Goals and objectives
2. Justification
3. Operating budget

(continued on next page)

(continued)
    4. Capital-needs report
    5. Cash forecast
    Each of these integral budget parts will be discussed in
detail in the sections that follow.

BUDGETING PROCESS

There are three phases of the budgeting process—*planning, preparation* and *control*. We'll discuss planning first.

■ Planning

A budget normally runs for one year. While this one-year budget provides the organization with a short-term plan of action, it's also a good idea to create a long-term budget for the next three to five years. Budgets are prepared by using previous experience and at the same time developing goals and objectives for the future. It's necessary to forecast activity for the next few years, and then predict how costs will respond to those activities and in what amounts.

The budget goals and objectives are a written expression of what the organization wants to accomplish in a specified period of time. They must be accepted by everyone involved, and they must again be S-M-A-R-T but in a slightly different way.

Specific: Be concise and to the point. Generalities and ambiguities will cause confusion and misinterpretation.

Measurable: Compliance must be determinable. If the actual results are vague, goals and objectives won't help.

Attainable: The goals must be within organizational reach or their inclusion in the plan will cause frustration and lethargy toward other goals.

Realistic: Similar to attainable. The goals and objectives must be a realistic part of the overall service mission and must be appropriate for the organization.

Tangible: The accomplishment of a specific goal or objective must be demonstrable. It must be something that the people in the organization can see or know.

As the group prepares budget goals and objectives, you should limit the scope of your ideas. It's wise not to try to accomplish everything at once. New ideas and programs should be phased in over a period of time. Some helpful hints are to identify specific targets with each objective and to limit the number of targets. If too many objectives are created, the organization's efforts will be diluted and its objectives may be left undone. Finally, deadlines should be set for each step of the plan. It's clearer to those responsible for the plan's implementation when they've been given a time frame within which to work.

■ Preparation

A budget gives the ambulance service and its staff members direction. Preparing a budget forces the organization to look at where it's been, where it is now and where it's going.

What do you need to prepare a budget? An involved governing body, administration and personnel. Members of the group have to be willing to invest some of themselves while preparing the budget. The organization must have a written statement of its goals and objectives. They must be clear and pertinent. It would be difficult, indeed, to write a financial plan for unclear or non-specific goals. It will be necessary for the budget group to have access to records of past operational activity as well as different expense and revenue account numbers. The chart of accounts is used to separate expenses into categories which can be measured and monitored. A sample of a chart of accounts is Appendix H. Finally, and most importantly, budget preparation takes *time*.

Budget justification demonstrates how numbers are calculated. Again, the budget is *not* a list of numbers, but a statement of ideas. The justification section of the budget correlates the numbers to the ideas. It contains the supporting documents and figures to show how expenses were computed. This validates any financial decisions and projections.

■ Components of the Operating Budget

The operating budget contains various figures and computations by which the organization will compare its future performance. The three parts of the operating budget include the statistics review, expense budget and revenue forecast.

Statistics Review. The *statistics review* is an accumulation of statistical data necessary to prepare the expense budget. There are numerous examples which may be included in the statistics and they vary considerably from service to service. The more statistical information available to the budget preparers, the more accurate the final document is apt to be. All information should be gathered which might help the budget writers make a better estimate of expenses and revenues. Besides financial information, the developers need data on the number of calls, types of calls, salaries, benefits, unit hours and maintenance costs. The history of the service's performance provides you with a basis to begin. It gives a picture of what has happened and where the service is now.

Preparing the Expense Budget. The next section of the operating budget is the *expense budget.* In the expense section, the projected expenses are itemized by specific category. For example, the phone charges are listed in one account, the rent in another, vehicle maintenance and salaries in others. Each associated area is subtotaled and the final total is computed. When determining the expenses, it's helpful to understand the different types of expenses. One of the easier ways to think of expenses is that they are fixed and variable. The fixed expenses are those costs that remain the same regardless of the level of activity of the service (for example, rent, salary, depreciation, etc.). The variable expenses vary with each unit of activity, such as medical supplies, ambulance linen, gasoline costs and so on. By understanding the way costs are affected by the activity of the service (number of runs), it makes it easier to predict the individual dollar amounts for each expense category.

Figure 3.1, a blank worksheet sample, demonstrates how the expense budget is organized. This worksheet is for preparing a yearly budget. The numbers for each expense account from the previous year are entered. Since budgets customarily are prepared a few months before the end of the fiscal year, the actual amount to be spent in each category for the entire year is estimated. This is called the annualized amount. The first column represents the annualized amount spent the previous year. The second column contains the budgeted amounts for the current year. This will indicate what areas were overbudgeted or underbudgeted. Programs or plans that were not accomplished last year might be seen in an overbudgeted category. Unexpected costs which were not planned for will be indicated in underbudgeted categories.

Figure 3.1   Budget Worksheet

Pg	Acct. #	Description	Est. Act. 19__	Budget 19__	Budget 19__

You can use the worksheet to fill out the new expense budget. Look at last year's activity and consider the new program costs which were developed in the justification section.

Estimating Expenses. This is where money management comes in. The manager watches the organization's money flow out. Much of the time it seems to go out faster than it comes in. What you have to do is make sure the company receives the greatest benefit for money spent. As with most industries that provide service to people, the EMS business is extremely labor intensive. In other words, the largest single expense will be for labor and benefits for labor. The section on personnel scheduling in Part 4 (page 201) discusses ways the service can increase its dollars' return spent on personnel.

While revenue generally comes from only a few sources, (patients, taxes, subscriptions, etc.), expenses can be divided into many categories. Other than personnel costs, there are expenses for medical supplies, equipment, vehicles, office expenses, licenses, accounting, legal services and a myriad of other groups. The competent manager controls and monitors expenses *closely*. If a service is under financial pressure, the board of directors usually doesn't ask that the staff reduce the number of emergency calls or the quality of care. They're instead likely to tell the director to curb expenses. Many times this is possible because every service has *some* waste. The trick in this uncomfortable situation is to trim fat without cutting meat from the bone. The unprepared manager may be in trouble if he can't support the necessary expenses in order to maintain quality service. The only way a manager can justify expenses is to be *in control* and completely *understand* the services's expenditures.

Preparing the Revenue Forecast. The *revenue budget* is next. Essentially, it's done the same way as the expense budget, but with fewer categories or accounts. For budgetary purposes, the patient revenues are determined by reducing the estimated gross-patient charges by the uncollectable percentage. Revenue is formally defined as the service's income from any source. There are two types of revenues for an ambulance service if it has no subsidiary businesses. There's a combined revenue derived from patient treatment and transport operations, commonly referred to as *patient revenue.* All other revenue from any other source is *non-operating revenue.* Non-operating revenues include subsidies, tax receipts, interest from savings and investments, training revenues, fund-raising income, donations, bequests and so on. By combining patient revenues with non-operating revenues and projected increases, it's possible to determine how much money the service will have for operating. Any projected increases in the charges should be listed on the revenue budget. The uncollectable percentage must be applied to those amounts as well. There are special characteristics, however, that need to be considered when charges are changed. First, if new charges or increases are added, it'll take 60 to 90 days before a significant increase will be seen on incoming payments. Another important point is that if the charges are raised significantly, there may be a corresponding decrease in the collection percentage. These effects are important to remember when the expense budget is balanced with the revenue budget.

■ Patient Revenue

A simple way to determine patient revenue is to multiply the total number of anticipated patient transports by the average patient charge. This isn't exact but generally comes close. The average patient charge is computed by dividing the total amount charged to patients over a specified time by the total number of patients transported in that same period of time.

Average-patient charge =
Total charges to patients ÷ Total patients transported

Projected gross revenue can then be calculated by multiplying the average patient charge by the total projected patient transports. Note: the total number of patients transported doesn't include either ambulance runs without a patient or non-billable charges.

Patient revenue =
Average-patient charge × Projected-patient transports

Once the gross-patient revenue is estimated, it's necessary to reduce that figure by the uncollectable amount. The uncollectable amount is easily determined by looking at the past performance of collections. A collection percentage can be determined by dividing the actual amount of payments received, during a specific period of time, by the gross patient charges for that same period.

Collection percentage =
(Total payments received ÷ Total charges to patients) × 100

The collection rate for most ambulance services varies between 55 and 80 percent. Population size, patient type and amount of the charges are all factors. Most significant, affecting actual collection rate, are a service's billing and collection practices. The collection percentage can be multiplied by the total patient charges to determine the total charges you can expect to collect. It's often clearer, however, to compute the amount of uncollectable charges. Subtract the collection percentage from 100 percent. That percentage is the uncollectable percentage. For example, if a service has a collection percentage of 75 percent, the uncollectable percentage is 25 percent.

The uncollectable percentage includes patients who can't or won't pay, as well as uncollected amounts due to agreements with third-party carriers such as Medicaid and Medicare. These are referred to as contractual allowances. Although they can significantly influence the collection rate, they must be included in the uncollectable percentage.

Services may find it advantageous to itemize revenue in detail—for example, routine transfers versus emergency runs. The procedures for calculating revenues are the same. Determine the average patient charge for each category. Multiply this by the number of transfers or emergencies in order to obtain gross revenue. Most difficult is determining the collection percentage for each transport category. Emergency patients have significantly poorer payment records than routine transports, and most small ambulance-service accounting systems can't separate the difference. The total collection percentage may produce inaccurate results for the two categories.

It's possible to provide more detail than the average patient charges. Each itemized charge can be identified. This gives the manager the advantage of seeing, for example, how much money an increase in the price of small bandages can generate over a year's time. He must, of course, remember to allow for uncollectables. The more information the manager has, the more likely the projections made will be accurate.

One more thing about projecting and understanding patient revenue. What if historical data are not available or if revenue patterns change? This can test even the most proficient service director who must rely on his experience and instinct. A new service doesn't have the advantage of experience, so how can you predict its number of calls? A rule of thumb, which is only marginally accurate, is that you can expect one emergency and one non-emergency call per day for each 10,000 people in your service area. Fortunately, it's rare that some form of historical information is not available from previous providers or other sources.

A change in activity can also affect revenue. Suppose a competing service moves into your service area. The new competitor can drastically alter your revenues, and the loss may be difficult to project. The organization's survival may depend on the manager's ability to both forecast the impact and respond to the change.

Establishing contracts with other health-care providers can provide additional sources of income. In many areas, contracts with hospitals, nursing homes, health-maintenance organizations, veteran's hospitals, state medical facilities, preferred-provider organizations, physicians and other providers have helped some services survive financially hard times. Other areas have neglected this source of income while an increasing number of publicly operated services are considering these attractive revenue sources.

In these contracts, the health-care provider usually agrees to use the service either exclusively or preferentially. In return, the service may provide a lower fixed rate. In highly competitive areas, these contractual relationships can give an ambulance service security as well as an edge over competitors.

Ambulance services can also contract to provide primary or backup services to communities. This might work well for smaller communities that can't support their own system. It might be worth exploring.

■ Non-operating Revenue

Non-operating revenue is that part of the services's income which is not attributed to patient charges. The most common non-patient revenues are subsidies. Subsidies are usually provided by a governmental entity to offset an ambulance service's losses. Taxes are the usual source. It might be a special tax earmarked for EMS, or it could come from city or county general revenues. Whenever taxes are used, some restrictions or accounting procedures may be mandated. Other organizations, such as hospitals, can also provide a subsidy to cover operating losses. The amount of the subsidy is usually fixed over a period of time.

There are many other revenue sources available if the manager is creative and open to new ideas. Volunteer fire departments have operated well for years by raising funds and seeking donations. Many ambulance services also rely on public good will for their existence. A well-planned and executed fund-raising program can provide a significant amount of revenue for the service. The possibilities are only limited by your imagination.

Non-profit services can also benefit from donations by stressing that such donations are often tax deductible. Donations of property, equipment and funds can be encouraged. In this case, it benefits the giver as well as the service. Bequests and endowments shouldn't be overlooked as a source of additional income. Colleges and hospitals have depended on the generosity of their patrons for years.

Subscriptions or membership programs may be the strongest alternative method for providing ambulance-service income. There are many types of membership programs throughout the country, some of which have enjoyed immense success. A membership program isn't easy to install. Publicity, promotion, record-keeping and administrative effort are required in large amounts for the successful implementation of a subscription service.

Some subscription services provide free use of the ambulance service to members. Others provide the service at a reduced cost. Many of the programs file and accept assignment for insurance benefits and don't require the members to pay out of their own pocket. There are programs which are offered only to senior citizens and many which are open to all. The costs vary considerably from program to program.

The design and implementation of a subscription program is complex. If your service decides that this type of revenue-producing program meets your needs, it's a good idea to review programs from other services before preparing your own program.

One source of income which is often overlooked by ambulance services is the creation of a subsidiary. Many private ambulance services have diversified into related and non-related businesses. Some ambulance services are providing full home health-care services, while others provide home respiratory-care services. Still others have medical equipment sales and rental services. Some owners are also dealers for emergency medical equipment or ambulance manufacturers. Still others have used their ambulance mechanics for outside maintenance services. Almost any type of business can be considered. Real estate, retail, nursing homes or other businesses might be the answer for a progressive service with an innovative governing body. Although the idea of creating a subsidiary to offset overhead may seem strange to public entities, there will be increasing pressure to diversify in the years ahead. In fact, that's why many city-affiliated fire departments have chosen to become involved in EMS.

Finally, the organization's revenues are going to depend largely on two things. First, patient-care income depends upon how well the service handles its accounts receivable. Effective billing policies and practices will enable the service to collect the largest amount of revenue possible. Billing and collection practices are covered in the next section of this part. Secondly, and just as important, is the quality of the service and its image. If the patient and the patient's family are satisfied with the treatment and demeanor of the field paramedics, the bill is more likely to be paid promptly and happily. Public support through donations and subscriptions is also determined by the level of customer and community satisfaction. Would you support a service for which you had little respect or confidence?

■ Capital-Needs Report

The *capital needs* is a listing of the major equipment purchases for the year. (See Figure 3.2) The items are probably not purchased each year but are one-time or infrequent purchases. These items are usually financed and usually not paid for outright. They have a life expectancy of years and are depreciated over their lifetime. The capital-equipment budget lists these items separately from the expense budget, because to include these irregular purchases in one of the expense accounts would artificially make it appear much larger than previous years. Instead, the cost of the items will appear in the expense budget as depreciation, payment on principal and interest expenses.

When developing capital equipment needs, it's helpful for the governing body, and others responsible for reviewing the budget, to

Figure 3.2   Capital-Needs Listing

CAPITAL NEEDS --1986			
CAPITAL EQUIPMENT	COST	LIFE/YRS	DEPRECIATION/YR
Ambulance	45,000	5	9,000
APCOR Radio	5,950	5	1,190
Hand Held Radios X 2	2,500	5	500
Mobile Radio	3,500	10	350
Office furniture & Computer equip.			
Computer memory expansion	1,500	5	300
Computer printer	2,700	5	540
Computer terminal	1,000	3	333
File Cabinet	800	10	80
	$62,950		$12,293

include the expected life of the equipment and the yearly depreciation costs. As a general rule, only that equipment which costs more than $500 is depreciated.

The service manager planning for the future should review the depreciation figure, and set funds aside in a separate equipment-replacement account. Then funds will be available when the equipment wears out.

■ Cash-Flow Forecast

The *cash-flow forecast* is the most difficult to determine. It's also one of the most important areas of which the manager must be aware. The cash-flow forecast helps determine if there will be enough money at the right time to pay for the costs of goals and objectives. The cash-flow analysis is usually done on a monthly basis. The projected expenses for each month are listed, and projected revenue is determined. Then these two figures are compared to make sure there will be enough cash to meet cash needs. This is a time-consuming process but is vitally necessary to ensure that there will be no unexpected cash-flow shortage.

Although many governmental service managers are not responsible for cash-flow forecasting, they should be encouraged to do so. This improves the EMS leader's credibility when dealing with municipal budget officers. Cash flow is their concern even if it's not the responsibility of the EMS manager.

■ Control

Once a budget document has been created, DON'T HIDE IT. Compare performance with the budget often, highlight variances and take action to correct any negative deviations. The control process uses various reports and information obtained throughout the year to compare the actual performance and financial situation with the budgeted projections. There are various ways to monitor the process. Some of the reports that may be used to monitor financial stability are the balance sheet, operating (profit/loss) statement, the statistical indicators report and other statistical reports. These reports must be complete, timely and accurate. Then corrective action can be taken sooner and more effectively.

CONCLUSION

EMS budgets come in many formats. There's no magic formula. But three important points must be re-emphasized. There must be COMMITMENT by the governing body and administration to the creation of the budget with organizational goals and objectives specified. The budget must be MONITORED. The actual performance must be compared with the projected performance indicated in the budget documents. And finally, the governing body and administration must be willing to TAKE ACTION quickly and effectively when deviations from the budget are discovered.

Billing and Collections

Overview

Every EMS and patient-transport service depends upon the money it receives. Even though this is an important factor, it's amazing how many services pay so little attention to billing and collections. One reason that so little progress is seen in this area is that many EMS services have evolved from, or are still, governmental or quasi-public agencies. It's well known that private industry places more emphasis than public services on getting the money.

This attitude is gradually changing as public money becomes scarce. Taxpayers are becoming increasingly concerned about government efficiency and how their monies are being spent. Services have to collect more revenue from patients rather than relying on public coffers. This has caused many managers to reevaluate their billing and collection system. What they're finding is a financial nightmare. While one public EMS service reported that last year they collected 13 percent of its receivables, others are discovering inadequate, inefficient and possibly illegal activities. This

(continued on next page)

(continued)

section is devoted to helping managers evaluate and change their billing and collection systems to maximize the money received from patient services. This has the long-term net effect of keeping the total cost for the service lower.

The secret to an outstanding billing and collection process is systemization. This means developing step-by-step procedures for handling patient accounts. A methodical process makes it possible to appropriately handle all types of accounts. This process is hard to describe—and even harder to accomplish. Proper handling of accounts is difficult and time consuming.

The billing and collection system should be a set of clearly defined, written procedures. It should eliminate all confusion and any questions about how particular accounts should be processed. The personnel involved should be well-oriented and trained in the procedures. Finally, there should be a clear audit trail.

The system described is designed around three principles. First, maximize income, then decrease the time it takes to receive the payments and finally handle income in the most cost-effective manner possible

The essential ingredients necessary to achieve maximum collections follow. Medical care must be of the highest quality as well as timely. Field and office personnel must be courteous, competent and professional at all times. Accurate and professional-looking invoices and statements should be provided to customers. Understand third-party reimbursement procedures, and make available any necessary assistance for filing or helping patients to file insurance claims. Establish a current accounts-receivable system, without backlogs of statements to be sent, claims to be filed, calls to be made or action to be taken on past-due accounts. Establish a means of measuring, documenting and analyzing so that managers can maintain control and determine the system's results. Develop and maintain *personal* attention and contact with your patients.

Most services don't have the clerical resources to file all

(continued on next page)

(continued)
types of insurances for their patients. The system we will describe is used by Criss Cross Ambulance Service (not their real name).

The patient is responsible for paying his bill. Criss Cross takes assignment on Medicare on a *claim-by-claim* basis. As a rule, they don't take assignment unless there's a definite reason to make an exception. Criss Cross neither accepts other insurance assignments nor files claims to other insurance companies. They will fill out an insurance claim, if requested, for a fee. Medicaid is accepted.

First, its necessary to discuss how controls are established to ensure all charges are documented and included in the paperwork sent to the billing office. The controls outlined in the section on inventory will help ensure charges are documented.

The second control check is the dispatch log. The dispatch log is a record of all calls the service responds to during a particular time or shift. Before a crew goes off duty, the communications staff, billing clerk, supervisor or other specified person should compare the log with the charge and patient information to determine that all paperwork and charges are complete for each run.

This information, including the log sheet, patient information, charges and run documentation, should be verified by the billing clerk(s). Next, verify patient information (name, address, phone, date of birth, insurance information, etc.) and any information necessary for filing insurance, Medicare or Medicaid, and check charges for accuracy and accountability.

Another person, such as a supervisor, should review the patient treatment, time spent on the scene and other run information to ensure that proper procedures and protocols were followed and to select runs for review and critique.

HANDLING VARIOUS ACCOUNTS

Now that the information has been verified, and missing or incorrect data have been collected or corrected, the trip is ready to be entered into the billing and collection system. Figures 3.3, 3.4, and 3.5 schematically show the flow of different patient accounts through the system.

The system is divided into three types of claims—private pay, Medicare and Medicaid. If a service were to file for all insurances, additional procedures would be needed. Patients who are responsible for filing their own claims are included in the private-pay category.

Accounts may move from one system to another. For example, if at first a patient is not listed as having Medicare, but at a later date you learn that the patient does indeed have Medicare, that account would flow from the private-pay system to the Medicare system. Thus, there aren't really three separate systems, but one billing and collection system, with different types of accounts handled in specific ways. For discussion and learning it's easier to understand and describe the system by breaking it into separate collection procedures.

Medicare and private payees should have an itemized statement mailed to the responsible party. This itemized invoice should be designed to include all the necessary information needed by the patient to file insurance forms. Because people are more likely to immediately pay an ambulance bill while the incident is fresh in their minds, the invoice should be mailed within 48 to 72 hours of the transport.

The second step is the same for all patients—personal and direct phone contact. A phone call performs a number of functions. Although not part of the actual collection process, it's used to determine the patient's satisfaction with the service and to offer assistance with processing claims. This courteous and friendly interaction should make the patient feel the ambulance service is genuinely and personally concerned about him. The patient or responsible party should be asked about the services received. Were they satisfied with the service? Were the crews helpful and timely? Do they have any suggestions? Is there any other way you can be of help to them? These types of questions serve two purposes. They break the ice with the patient and exhibit a sincere desire to know whether the patient was satisfied with the service. They also help measure the performance

Figure 3.3 Private-Payee Billing Diagram

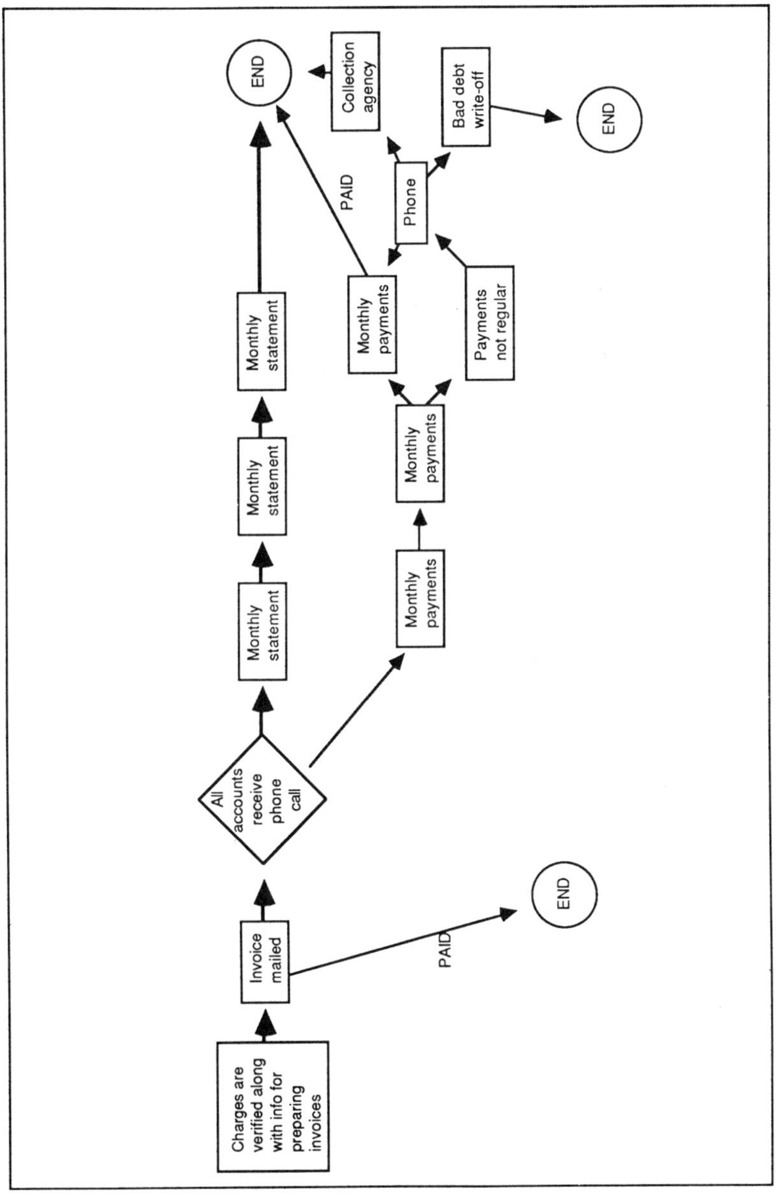

Figure 3.4 Medicare Billing Diagram

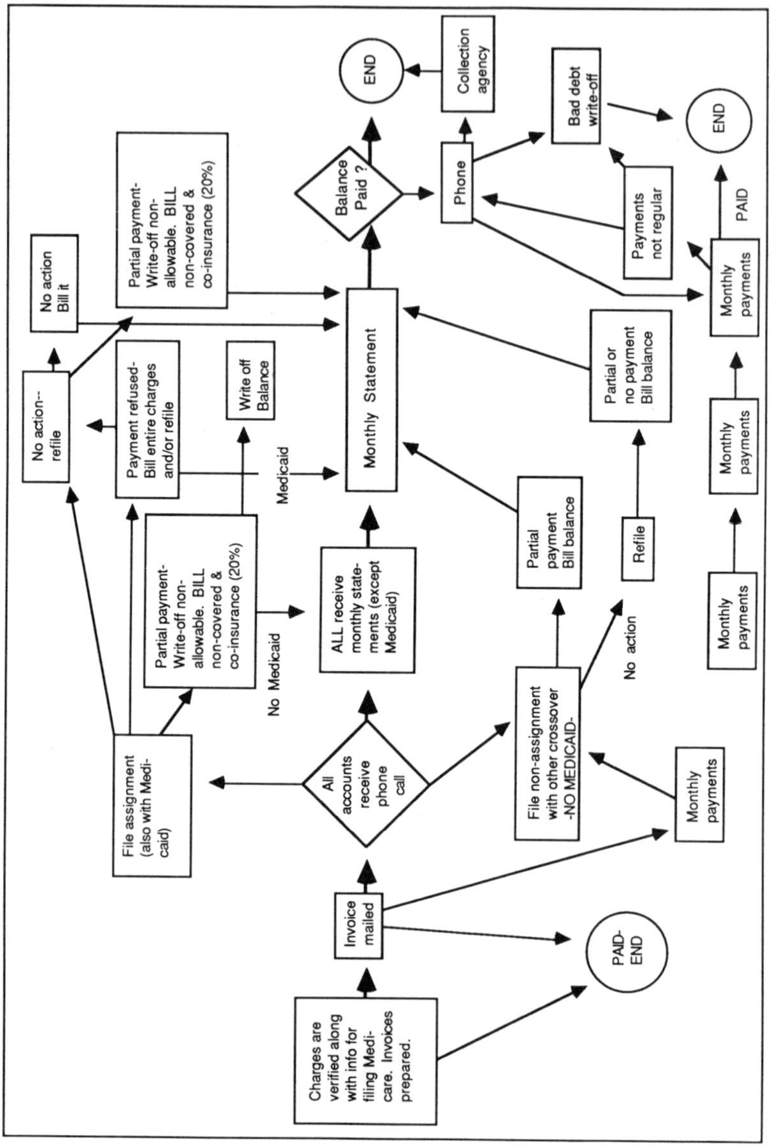

Figure 3.5   Medicaid Billing Diagram

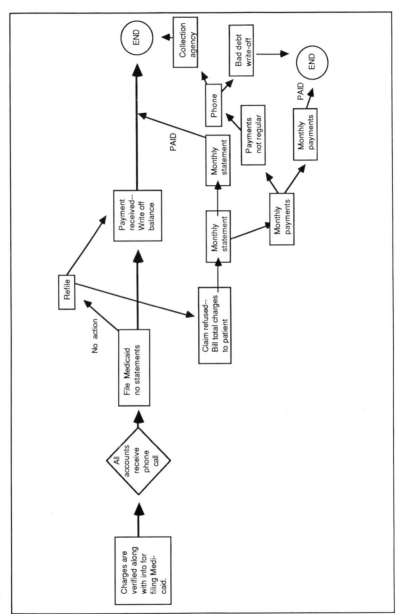

of the involved field personnel to determine how well they were received by the patient and his family.

After breaking the ice, you can gather account information about insurance and discuss other missing items. Again, the emphasis should be on helping the patient and his family during this trying time. This is a good time to discuss the service's policies on insurance assignment, Medicare filing, and so on.

Three questions should be answered during this short conversation. Was the patient satisfied with the service? How should the account be handled by the service's billing and collection system (for example, Medicare, Medicaid, private pay)? Is there anything unique about the patient's situation which could effect how the account will be handled?

When you call is important. Ideally, this conversation should take place prior to the patient receiving his first statement. It often seems that how satisfied a patient is with the service is inversely proportionate to the amount of the bill. A more objective opinion is often received before the patient is billed. This may eliminate complaints about the service later on.

All three ways of dealing with accounts are based on a 90-day maximum cycle. If the service doesn't receive payment within 90 days, the possibility of being paid drastically decreases. Every effort should be made to collect payment as soon as possible.

■ Private-Pay accounts

After phone contact, private-pay accounts essentially follow three paths. (1) The account is paid promptly. (It's often advantageous to offer a discount—say 10 percent—to those patients who pay their accounts in full within 30 days.) (2) The patient makes a partial payment. (3) No action takes place.

If the account is paid in full, no further action is needed unless the patient requests assistance in filing insurance claims. This is the ideal way for an account to be cleared.

The patient may begin making payments. Many people have limited financial resources, especially after a medical problem that necessitated ambulance transport. As long as they pay regularly, at least monthly, patients should be supported in their paying efforts. Some money is better than no money! Their accounts should be reviewed periodically to make sure they aren't slipping on their agreed-upon payments. Send monthly or bi-monthly statements as reminders. Eventually, most of these accounts will be paid in full.

No action will take place on some accounts. These accounts need special attention. Write and phone these customers after 30 days to remind them of their account status. This direct contact may initiate payment on inactive accounts.

If an account goes 65 to 70 days with no payment or adequate explanation, take firmer action. Write, stating that the account will be turned over to a collection agency or legal representative. Then call, clearly stating that the account can no longer be ignored and that action will be taken within a specified time. Be sure that all activities at this point fall within acceptable collection practices. These practices are governed by federal and state laws and should be reviewed by the service's attorney. This type of effort is also required on accounts to which previous payments were made but which have been inactive for 45 days.

Finally, if no money or adequate plan for payment is received, it will be necessary to take final action. Depending upon the patient's economic situation and effort, the account should either be turned over to a collection agency or written off as a charity case.

■ Medicare accounts

The itemized statement and phone call are initially directed toward the patient or responsible party. If the patient is economically depressed, a likely non-payer of debts or on Medicaid, it'll probably be best to file assignment for Medicare or Medicaid.

Sometimes, full or partial payment will be made. If payment is made, no other action is needed except filing non-assignment for the patient so Medicare will reimburse part of the out-of-pocket money. Often, patients will apply their total reimbursement checks to the account.

All patients, except those with Medicaid, should receive regular statements. This tells a patient what the current status of his account is. If a patient pays on a Medicare-assignment account, and payment is made by Medicare, it will be necessary to reimburse the patient any money he previously paid to the service.

■ Assignment accounts

If no activity occurs within 60 days of filing a claim, the claim should be re-filed with the Medicare carrier. When payment is received, *non-covered* items, the 20 percent co-payment, and any remaining annual deductible should be billed to the patient. If Medicaid is involved, write off the remaining balance as a contractual allowance for Medicaid. Also write off any non-allowed charges to Medicare allowances.

Sometimes the claim will be denied. In that case, the full charges should be billed to the patient.

■ Non-assignment accounts

If the patient notifies the service that nothing has been received from Medicare 60 days after the claim has been filed, the service should re-file with the carrier. Otherwise, the account is handled as a private-pay account, with regular statements mailed indicating payments as they occur. If there's no further activity after another 30 days, other collection procedures should be used (for example, reminder letters, phone calls, pre-collection letters and finally, a collection agency).

■ Medicaid

Medicaid regulations are generally strict. It's important these accounts are handled properly. If Medicaid is filed, or if it's known that the patient has Medicaid, the service is forbidden to bill the patient or accept payments on the account.

Once Medicaid is filed, don't send statements to the patient. If a Medicaid payment isn't received within 60 to 90 days (it usually takes longer than Medicare), the claim should be re-filed. When a payment is received from Medicaid, the remaining balance *must* be written off to Medicaid contractual allowances.

The other possibility is that the claim may be denied. In that case, bill the patient directly for all charges. The rest of the account should be similar to the private-pay system. The only difference is that the unpaid accounts will probably be written off to charity rather than turned over to the collection agency.

FOOTNOTES

This discussion has briefly demonstrated the flow, and activity, of various types of accounts through a billing and collection system.

There are a few related points which should now be presented.

Returned mail: Patient accounts with incorrect or incomplete information, such as wrong addresses or patient names, need early action. If you can't obtain accurate information from hospitals or by other means and it's impossible to reach the patient or responsible party, these accounts should be traced or turned over to a collection agency as soon as possible. The sooner the agency can start its investigation, the better the results.

Collection agency: Collection agencies are like any other business. Some are more efficient and effective than others. In selecting a collection agency, evaluate its past experience, especially regarding medically related accounts. It's also possible to negotiate a better percentage for the service with these agencies. Don't just accept the first offer. Try for a better deal. Another strategy is to split similar accounts into two different agencies to determine which one brings a higher return.

Bankruptcy: Often, if you notify the service that a patient has declared bankruptcy, the remainder of that patient's account will be written off to charity or as a bad debt.

Probate: A deceased patient's estate can be tied up in probate for a considerable period of time. Keep these accounts open, and follow all proper procedures for recovery of funds through probate.

Liens: Hospitals have, for a long time, filed liens with insurance companies for auto-accident victims. This assures them of the best possible recovery of funds from insurance companies. Since EMS is *also* health-care related, it may be possible for ambulance services to use such lien laws to their advantage. Research this with your service's legal advisor to evaluate the possibility of including it in the service's procedures.

Statements: How often should you send statements? The answer to this frequently asked question, of course, varies with the resources available to the service. Statements should be sent at least once a month. Many people are paid twice a month—at the middle and end. It's good practice to send statements so they arrive a few days before payday when the patient is most likely to be paying his bills.

Over-90-day reviews: The only way a system can effectively work is with close monitoring. At least once a month, review every account that's over 90 days old. This review determines what is happening with each account and what action, if any, is necessary. What may be needed is a phone call, to write it off, turn it over to a collection agency, to re-file insurance, and so on.

Computerization: You may find your service needs computerization of accounts receivable. Some systems increase the efficiency and effectiveness of billing and collections. Selecting a computer system for the ambulance service can be a difficult, if not overwhelming, responsibility for the manager. Often, the selected system has many flaws, especially if it's not specifically designed for ambulance services. Ambulance accounts-receivable systems come in three basic varieties.

(1) Packaged system: Although these generic systems may be generally designed for ambulance services, managers may find it frustrating that they don't meet the particular needs of their service.

(2) Fully customized: This software is usually a basic EMS computerized medical-billing system, modified by consultants to meet specific service requirements.

(3) Home-grown: This type of system usually causes the most frustration and, in the end, may be the most expensive when one considers time. It's usually developed by a whiz-kid programmer or by the manager. These systems are generally replaced within six to 12 months.

Computerizing accounts receivable can significantly improve cash flow. Most services underestimate both the initial cost and the ongoing maintenance and programming costs for computers. Even small services, however, should seriously consider computers. Regardless of whether the billing and collection system is manual or computerized, it will require increased attention by EMS managers of the future.

ACCOUNTING NEEDS

Now that money is coming in, how do you handle it? Good solid accounting practices are a must. Security and efficiency depend on it. Accountability means accounting for every dollar that flows in and out of the organization, as well as what happens to it while in the organization's hands. This process involves bookkeeping and management. The purpose is to ensure no money escapes, either intentionally or accidentally, and that every penny is used to the best benefit of the organization.

If you've ever seen a report from an accounting firm, the phrase "according to generally accepted accounting practices" probably rings a bell. Accounting and bookkeeping are well-established and accepted business disciplines because they document and monitor the flow of money. The ambulance business is a complex industry. The lack of sound financial practices will invariably lead to problems. These problems may surface as theft or embezzlement, but will more likely result in the service having a money crisis. Bankruptcy and service shut-downs are not uncommon.

It's not our intention to offer a class in accounting. Instead, we want to expose managers to the terms and practices that should be used. Frankly, we recommend that services use a competent, qualified accountant to develop a system of controls for the organization. In the public sector, there may be specialists within a local governmental unit who can be temporarily assigned to the service to help with such a project. The accountant's role is more than simply providing monthly, quarterly or yearly financial reports or a bookkeeping service. He's to assist in designing and implementing a complete system for bookkeeping and financial monitoring. An accountant can also explain and train administrative personnel in the use of the system, and teach them how they can help make better decisions about funds entrusted to the service.

Remember—a good accounting system will provide protection from the mishandling of money, eliminate mistakes and provide the director and governing body with the information necessary to monitor the financial performance of the organization.

There are a number of packaged systems that provide basic bookkeeping, such as daily income reports, expense reports and monthly reports, and include checks to prevent errors in matching income with deposits. These business systems, coupled with a double-entry bookkeeping system, are usually sufficient to provide the essentials. Computerized systems are also available for almost any size service. Whatever type of accounting system you use, it's still necessary to support the system with good money-handling policies. Who can receive money? Who records payments to patient accounts? Who signs checks, makes deposits, reconciles bank statements and prepares the payroll? These are all questions which need to be answered by the service's procedures. Double checking and monitoring are important when it comes to money. Other decisions about collection policies, use of credit cards, purchasing practices and inventory control will impact the service's financial picture. The accountant can assist in the development of these procedures to effectively monitor a service's cash flow and streamline its efficiency.

Third-Party Reimbursements— Medicare, Medicaid and Other Players

Overview

A pivotal factor in the success of an ambulance operation is the amount of revenue generated from patient services. This revenue is primarily influenced by the reimbursement practices of various health insurers including Medicare, Medicaid, private insurance firms and Workmen's Compensation. It's been said that over 80 percent of all Americans are covered by some form of health and accident insurance. The ambulance manager's task, when appropriate, is to capture these funds for the provision of prehospital care and medical transportation. This lowers the actual direct cost for both user and taxpayer.

There are hundreds of companies which provide health insurance, but the majority of the patients transported by ambulance have Medicare, Medicaid, Blue Shield or a

(continued on next page)

(continued)
combination of the three. This section's focus will be on
Medicare and Medicaid since most services receive a
significant amount of income from these two sources and
understand them the least.

HISTORY

Both Medicare and Medicaid went into effect in 1966 as a result
of President Johnson's Great Society Program. Medicare provides
federally funded government health insurance for people 65 years of
age and older. Medicare is actually two programs—hospital insurance
funded through the Federal Hospital Insurance Trust Fund (Part A
of Medicare) and medical insurance funded through the Federal
Supplementary Insurance Trust Fund (Part B of Medicare). Medicare
regulations are extremely complex. Certain types of care are only
covered under Part A while other types are only covered under Part
B. For example, Part A helps pay for inpatient hospital care and
inpatient care in a skilled nursing facility. Part B covers ambulance
services, doctors' services, outpatient hospital care and health services
and supplies not covered by Part A. Unless the provided ambulance
service is considered a department of a hospital, medical
transportation services are covered under Part B. Medicare coverage
is available only after the appropriate medical-necessity guidelines are
met. Unless ambulance-service managers understand entitlement and
its qualifications, they cannot secure the maximum benefits a patient
may be able to receive.

Medicaid is a combined federal-state program with the federal
government contributing a portion of the total funds required. The
Medicaid program is administered by individual states to provide
medical care for those people whose low incomes would otherwise
prevent them from being cared for. These individuals are usually
referred to as medically indigent. Since each state defines indigent
differently, there are wide variations in state programs. Unlike
Medicare, Medicaid is intended to cover all medical needs of the
indigent regardless of age. Although most states have medical-
transportation benefits available for its recipients, the Medicaid

program has been the victim of the budget ax in recent years. Because of these cutbacks, Medicaid usually reimburses ambulance services far below their service costs.

MEDICARE

First, we'll examine Medicare. To do so, it's important to understand some terminology. Some of these terms are defined in the glossary in the appendix. However, several terms need to be defined now.

Carrier. A commercial insurance firm or Blue Shield plan administering Part B of Medicare.

Beneficiary. The patient receiving the service or supply who is an eligible participant in the Medicare program.

Provider. An ambulance service, physician or supplier who is an eligible and bona-fide member of the Medicare plan as determined by the carrier through an application and approval process.

Co-insurance. A provision by which the patient must pay for a portion of his or her medical expenses. This refers to the 20 percent of reasonable charges for which the Medicare beneficiary is responsible after the deductible has been met.

There may be a single carrier or multiple carriers in each state. Each carrier is responsible for a specified region and all of the providers in that region file with that carrier. The problem is that each carrier formulates many of its own policies. Even though the federal government has specific guidelines for *all* carriers, each carrier interprets them differently so that reimbursement practices vary.

The carrier provides the ambulance service with its specific set of guidelines for obtaining reimbursement for services. The Medicare manual will describe in detail how to fill out each claim and instruct on what information is necessary.

Accuracy is important. Therefore, submit Medicare claims with a 98 percent level of accuracy in mind. Each time a claim is improperly completed, it delays reimbursement and adds expenses for rehandling time.

Covered services. Covered services are those medical and health services covered under Medicare Part B. Certain field procedures are covered while others may not be. When a payment is received from the Medicare carrier for services, the non-covered services and amounts are listed. These non-covered services can be billed directly to the patient as a total charge.

Types of Covered Transports. Not all ambulance transports are covered under Medicare Part B. All carriers have guidelines that determine if a transport is covered. Some of the transports that are covered follow.

1. Transport from an injury scene to the closest hospital.
2. Transport from hospital to hospital *if* the discharging hospital does not have the appropriate medical services required for the patient's condition.
3. Transport from a hospital to a skilled nursing home *if, and only if,* medical necessity can be established and the home is near the institution.
4. Transport from a skilled nursing home to a hospital to a skilled nursing home if the pickup point is within the service area of the destination and the service is determined to be medically necessary.
5. Transport from a hospital to a hospice center if the hospice center is determined by the carrier to be the best medically suited facility for the patient's condition.

Some of these covered transports may be denied if it's determined the trip was not medically necessary or if the patient could have been transported by other means—even if the other means of transportation were not available to the patient. Many other claims are rejected because of poor documentation.

Non-covered Transports. Certain transports aren't covered by Medicare.

1. Transport from a skilled nursing home to an airport or any other non-medical destination.
2. Transport from a hospital to a physician's office, from a skilled nursing home to a physician's office or from a home to a physician's office. Medicare will not cover transport to a physician's office unless it's medically necessary to stop en route to a hospital. A manager should check this with the carrier, however, because recent interpretations indicate that carriers have been paying for some specific physician trips when the procedure could be done less expensively than in a hospital.

3. Transport to a free-standing medical facility.
4. Long-distance transport by ground ambulance.
5. Transport from hospital to hospital if the carrier has determined the discharging hospital to be medically suitable for the patient's condition, regardless of whether or not the patient's physician is on staff at the discharging hospital.
6. Transport for convenience of patient or family.
7. Transport from home to a skilled nursing facility (SNF), or from a SNF to home.

There are other times when transport is unlikely to be covered but is considered on an individual basis by the carrier. Transport from a hospital to the patient's home is often denied. The carrier may feel that if the patient is well enough to be discharged, the patient should be able to travel by other means. Also, many transports from a skilled nursing home and back are considered medically unnecessary and, therefore, denied.

SHOULD WE ACCEPT ASSIGNMENT?

There are two ways to file a Medicare claim—for assignment or for non-assignment. If the service accepts assignment on a Medicare claim, that service then agrees to accept the Medicare allowable charges as payment in full for the service.

For example, a $200 ambulance bill is submitted to Medicare. The carrier determines (from its magic formulas) that all the charges are covered. They also determine that the allowable charges for the services are $140. If the service accepted assignment on this claim, the provider would be eligible to receive 80 percent of the allowable charges, or $112, from the Medicare carrier. In addition, the service could then bill the patient for the remaining 20 percent of the claim which in this case would be $28. The balance of $60 would have to be written off to Medicare contractual allowances. The patient cannot be billed for any part of the non-allowed charges by the carrier.

There are a few more peculiarities and rules when filing for assignment. If the service accepts an assignment, the service receives payment directly from the carrier. If the deductible has not yet been met by the patient, the deductible bill is then directly billable to the patient. Once you submit an assigned claim, you can't change it before the claim is paid. Even if the ambulance service files for assignment, the service can bill *non-covered* services to the patient at full charge. (In the example above all, the charges were covered, so this didn't apply.) Many services miss this step and, therefore, an opportunity to increase their revenue. The beneficiary is responsible for the co-payment amount as well as the annual deductible that hasn't been met—*plus* any non-covered services.

Many ambulance services receive requests from Medicare to sign provider agreements to accept assignment. This agreement says the service will accept what Medicare pays on the claim as payment *in full* except for the annual deductible which will remain the beneficiary's responsibility. It also says the service will accept assignment on *all* Medicare claims. There's no penalty for those ambulance services that don't sign the agreement. It's important that the manager carefully determine the impact of signing such an agreement before doing so. It may not be in the service's best financial interest.

When filing assignment, the service, with the beneficiary's approval, applies directly to Medicare for reimbursement. This signifies an agreement by the service to accept the carrier's determination of reasonable charges for its services. The beneficiary is then responsible only for the deductible plus 20 percent of the balance of the reasonable charge.

The other option for the service is to file non-assignment. In this case, the beneficiary files the claim with the carrier and directly receives the reimbursement. The provider gives the patient an itemized statement and diagnosis to file. Many ambulance services file the non-assignment claim form for the patient. That's the reason the run report has a block for the patient's signature authorizing the service to file. In this case, however, the reimbursement check from the carrier will go directly to the patient.

If a non-assignment claim is filed, the service can bill the *entire service charge* to the patient, often collecting the total bill before the Medicare claim is processed. The service is not bound by any agreement with Medicare to accept what the carrier has deemed to be reasonable charges for the services provided. Let's look again at our example of the $200 ambulance bill. In the case of non-assignment, the entire $200 bill is rendered to the patient for payment. The patient can submit a claim to the carrier and receive a reimbursement of $112. In this way, no matter what Medicare pays, the patient is responsible for the entire $200 bill for the service.

■ Why non-assignment may be better

There are many arguments for filing non-assignment. Unfortunately, many aren't based on the issues. It should be emphasized that *services can decide assignment status on a claim-by-claim basis*. Let's return to our example. If the service bills the patient $200 for services rendered and makes diligent attempts to collect over a 60- to 90-day pay period, but is unsuccessful, it can still file for assignment and receive the $112 from Medicare. It then tries to collect the $28 from the patient once the claim is paid by Medicare. One word of caution: this will reduced the timeliness of payment from Medicare. It's more appropriate to file non-assignment or assignment as soon as possible after the date of service. There are two exceptions to this. One is if the service has previously signed a Medicare Provider Assignment Agreement. The second is if Medicaid is filed (medi/medi), then assignment on Medicare is required.

Deciding on a claim-by-claim basis eliminates many of the arguments for accepting assignment on all claims. One argument frequently heard is "If the patient gets the money, we'll never see it." This is a valid argument in some cases, but it's more likely a reflection on the service's billing and collection practices. Competent billing personnel and an efficient billing system, whether manual or computerized, will identify many of the bad risks prior to filing. If not, the next time this patient who has beaten the service out of its money requires care, the service can file the claim-assignment to assure that the funds come directly to the service.

In fairness to those who advocate accepting assignment on all medicare patients, this non-assignment approach does require a more sophisticated billing system. However, most services which have done a cost-benefit analysis indicate that it's well worth the investment when one considers the net return to the organization.

Many publicly operated services historically filed for assignment on a routine basis to simplify the billing process. Times are changing and these services are searching for additional revenue. These same services may be able to significantly increase their reimbursements by improving their billing systems.

■ Reasonable-charge determinations

If the reasonable charges allowed by Medicare carriers were actually reasonable and uniform, assignment wouldn't be a problem.

Unfortunately, this isn't the case. The means by which the reasonable charges are calculated are inherently inequitable. Many consider them downright unfair. In many cases, it results in an allowable charge that is far below the cost of the service.

The procedure is complex. Here's an oversimplified explanation. All services are placed in a region for comparison with other services. This isn't necessarily a geographic region. Each item or service is tallied with the amount for each ambulance service in the region. A scale is determined, with the highest charges for each item placed at 100 percent. The carrier then determines the 75th percentile using a series of averages. This is the amount which is determined reasonable, and the carrier reimburses to all services in the region 80 percent of this amount, or 80 percent of the actual charges—whichever is lower.

All services in the region are included in the development of this screen. It makes no difference to the carrier that the reason many publicly operated service charges are artificially lower is because of local tax subsidization and that their *true cost* for providing the service may be as high as any of the other services. In this way, the service that charges $35 per trip ("because we don't want high fees") is actually undermining the reimbursement for the patients of all the other services in that region. Those patients are being charged a fee that more closely represents the cost to provide the service. Now, if you don't understand the "profile-smasher" dilemma, re-read the last two paragraphs.

Deciding whether or not to accept assignment should be done with attention to costs and the amount the service receives from Medicare. It's important that the patient's out-of-pocket cost is reasonable. If you don't want to cut off your nose to spite your face, it's also necessary to charge near the actual cost of providing service.

Several things are helpful in this decision-making process. They can be obtained from your Medicare carrier. First is a printout of your service's charge mix and the allowable rate for each charge. This shows exactly how much the carrier allows for each item and what you'll be reimbursed. If you decide to raise a charge, however, remember that the carrier will only re-evaluate charges once a year. Second is a list of current reasonable charges for your region. This shows the range of charges within the region. It will help you determine what is a reasonable charge for each item and will help you evaluate the adequacy of your service's charges. For example, if Criss Cross Ambulance Service charges $15 to monitor a patient, the allowable charge is $50, and they receive $12 for the procedure. If Goodwill Ambulance charges $50, they receive $40 for the same procedure that Criss Cross received for $12. Remember, 80 percent of allowable or 80 percent of the actual charge—whichever is lower. Another useful strategy is to review what items or services you charge separately for and which you include in the base rate. If the carrier allows a charge for defibrillation, for example, and your service doesn't charge for that procedure, you could be missing much needed revenue.

■ Confusion about interhospital transfers

Transportation from hospital to hospital or to another freestanding medical facility and return for specialized diagnostic or therapeutic services not available in the inpatient's hospital must be billed to the sending hospital. Simply stated, if the Medicare beneficiary remains an inpatient at one hospital and is transported somewhere else for tests or treatment, the hospital, not the patient, must be billed. Hospitals billed for these services are required to pay the provider of the service. It's acceptable to set a discounted rate with hospitals for these transports. In any event, it's in the service's best interest to establish contractual relationships with hospitals. This policy does *not* cover transports for admission, transfers between a hospital and the patient's home or transfers between hospitals and skilled nursing homes.

■ Medical necessity

It's impossible to detail how to fill out each type of claim form and the specific codings used. A manual for ambulance providers is available from the carrier with step-by-step instructions.

The *critical* aspect of submitting a claim, which determines whether or not the claim will be paid, is the presumptive medical diagnostic information decided by the technician. This proves to the carrier that the patient could not have traveled any other way. This is determined by the patient's need for medical care.

IMPROVED DOCUMENTATION EQUALS IMPROVED REIMBURSEMENT

Many times, claims are denied solely because of semantics. A heart condition does not, by itself, justify ambulance transportation, while an acute MI does. The wording and completeness of the diagnostic information is essential to determine payment.

Some acceptable and unacceptable examples of diagnoses are listed below. They're presented here to illustrate why ambulance personnel must complete the run-report form completely and accurately. We're not suggesting that field employees write creative reports to artificially increase reimbursement for services rendered. It should be noted, however, that many services claim that when employees are trained in report writing, and documentation improves, there is a significant effect on reimbursements.

Some acceptable diagnoses include unconsciousness, shock or comatose, cardiac arrest, acute or complete stroke (CVA), acute myocardial infarction (AMI) and convulsions. Also acceptable is if the patient requires oxygen, IV maintenance ECG monitoring or other emergency care or treatment. If the patient is confined to a bed, unable to walk and can be moved only by a stretcher, has a spinal or back injury or needs restraining en route, you can consider the diagnosis acceptable.

Unacceptable diagnoses, on the other hand, include intoxication, behaviorally disturbed, possible GI bleeding (sometimes acceptable depending on severity), fractured arm, nausea or vomiting or a heart condition with no further explanation. Other diagnoses in this category are doctor-ordered ambulance transports, if the patient is dead prior to call for an ambulance (claim acceptable if the patient dies en route to hospital), severe illness with no further explanation, patient too sick to walk with no further explanation and a patient requiring dialysis treatment (unless significant diagnostic information is supplied which proves that ambulance transport is medically necessary in *each* case).

Remember, accurate and complete diagnostic information and treatment information results in fewer claims being denied as medically unnecessary.

MEDICAID

Since Medicaid is administered by individual states, the rules and regulations are not universal. As with Medicare, the service must apply to the state for approval as a provider. Medicaid forms are standardized, but the state may require various supporting documentation, including copies of patient-care forms, physician's medical-necessity statements and other documents.

The amount of money which Medicaid progams reimburse providers varies widely from one program to another. The amount may be fixed, such as $50 per transport, or it may be tied to what is allowed by Medicare. Medicaid programs are often more restrictive than Medicare regarding which transports are approved. Reimbursement may be limited to only life-threatening emergencies or other specific criteria.

For example, in the state of Missouri, the reimbursement from *Medicaid only* applies to emergency transports. A fixed amount is paid for each call (in 1987 it was $50). A limited number of add-on procedures or supplies are also covered. A copy of the Missouri State Ambulance Run Report is required to accompany the Medicaid claim form. Each Medicaid claim is reviewed by a physician to determine the medical necessity of ambulance transportation. Therefore, the documentation and completeness of the patient diagnostic and treatment information is of utmost importance.

Even though Medicaid may pay only a small portion of ambulance service costs, it shouldn't be overlooked as a source of revenue. The participants in Medicaid programs have *already* met the requirements which determine they are unable to pay for medical care. This pre-screening should indicate to the manager that he should get all available funds to help cover the service's cost—in this case Medicaid.

By filing a Medicaid claim, the ambulance service agrees to accept the Medicaid reimbursement as *payment in full* for services provided. The service is not allowed to bill the patient if Medicaid is filed. If a Medicaid claim is denied or the person isn't covered by Medicaid, the patient can be billed for the full charges. However, the collection percentage on these accounts will be low. Because the Medicaid patient is poor, collecting money on his accounts should be handled with compassion. Many of these accounts will eventually be written off to charity.

FILING A CLAIM

Honest-claim filing. We've all heard about those doctors or health-care providers who have been charged with Medicare or Medicaid fraud. To counteract such practices, agencies have established programs and procedures to prevent and discover fraud. As an EMS manager, be aware of intentional wrongdoings, and make sure the service allows no accidental errors or oversights.

Medicare can only be filed with permission from the beneficiary, both for assignment and non-assignment. This is why it's necessary for the patient to sign either a Medicare form or other release form. The ambulance manager must ensure that signatures are collected before filing Medicare or other insurance claims.

Keep a Medicare and Medicaid log. It will help you keep track of all claims filed and their status.

Other insurance. Insurance companies can be billed directly for services rendered to their clients. Most hospitals file insurance claims for patients. Generally, the hospitals are directly paid by the companies. Ambulance services can also follow this policy, but there are numerous insurance companies and many require individual forms. Even though this policy may increase collections, the time and increased personnel involved may offset the additional income. This should be carefully evaluated before deciding which procedure to use.

The ambulance company can also send an itemized bill directly to the patient. It's then the patient's reponsibility to file with his or her insurance company or companies.

Crossover. Many Medicare carriers have developed a crossover system with other insurance companies such as Medicaid, Blue Cross or Blue Shield. In such cases, only one claim is filed with Medicare. The information and account number for the crossover insurance companies are included on the claim. After the Medicare carrier acts on the claim, it transfers it to the appropriate reimbursement agencies for consideration. This process eliminates the necessity of filing multiple claims. Be sure you know what crossovers are available to your carrier.

Note that third-party reimbursement is complicated. But an efficient system of handling insurance claims can dramatically increase the revenue generated from patient services. All aspects of the billing and collection system should be thoroughly evaluated to make sure needed dollars are not slipping through the cracks.

C A S E   S T U D Y   # 5

Medicare

John's concerned. For four hours last night he poured over these same figures and now still can't see what's gone wrong. As executive director of Ambassador Ambulance Service, he's worked hard to balance revenues with expenses. The numbers he presented to the board yesterday weren't good—both receipts and collection rates have gradually declined over the last six months. Although he isolated the main problem area last night—Medicare reimbursement—he still can't understand why Medicare is paying less and why payment seems to be slower. Examining possibilities, John determines the following:

—There's been no increase in charges which would cause Medicare to reimburse a smaller percentage of the charges.
—There's been no change in the allowable rate.
—No new charges or procedures have been added to the service's bills.
—The number of transported Medicare patients has remained constant.
—Assignment policies are the same and there's been no change in Medicare deductible.
—Medicare claims are being sent out promptly.

John shakes his head. Everything seems to be the same, so why has the collection rate decreased? He decides to talk to Bonnie, his office manager. Bonnie started with Ambassador five years ago. She's been fantastic. The office has never been more organized. Productivity is high and, at the same time, everyone seems to like her.

"Bonnie, we seem to have a problem, and I'd like your input."

John explains the situation of decreasing collection percentage from Medicare.

"That's easy, those people at the Medicare carrier's office are just trying to hold on to their money, says Bonnie. "It's how the government tries to save money. They deny a lot more claims and consistently hassle us about documentation."

"Bonnie, I don't understand. The money isn't the carrier's, its money for the beneficiaries. The carriers are required to reimburse for covered services. What's happened to change it all?"

"Well, nine months ago the carrier changed from Itna National to Purple Cross. When Itna handled the claims, we had no problems. We could work with those people. These people at Purple Cross just don't know what they're doing, and every time I call them all I get is the runaround."

"Any changes in how we file Medicare with the new carrier?"

"That's just it! We're doing everything *exactly* the same way as before. We're even using Itna's provider manual..."

John pauses. "I still don't understand why we aren't getting reimbursed like before."

"I don't either. Same forms, same coding, same procedures. It's just that those new people at Purple Cross are denying more claims. They don't respond the way Itna did. *Those* people just don't want to turn loose of their money. They just want to make life difficult for us."

Bonnie looks at John's smile, then reflects on what she's just said. "It's my attitude toward the new carrier, isn't it? I haven't built a good rapport, and I've established an adversarial relationship."

"So, Bonnie, what's the plan?"

"Well, now it's obvious. We have a new carrier with new people and new rules. I've worked by the old rules and that's not appropriate. I haven't made the effort to get to know any of the new carrier people. I've got to set up a specific action plan to change that."

"Such as?" John asks.

"First, I'll set up an appointment with the provider-relations representative for week after next. In the meantime, I'll ask them to send me their provider's manual. Then, I'll evaluate every claim denial and request we've received during the last three months. That way I can better understand what we haven't been doing according to their rules."

"What are you going to do at the carrier's office?"

"I'm going to meet the people—put names to faces, or I should say names to voices. I'll ask what we can do to make their job easier. I'll make an effort to meet the claims processor, or processors, who work on our claims. They should have a good idea what we should do to make processing more efficient. I think I'll even invite them to visit our office. It might give them an idea of how difficult *our* job is, too. It'd also be nice for Beth and Kate to meet the people they talk to on the phone. I'll take them with me to Purple Cross office and invite their people to see an ambulance operation."

"Good plan. Let me know how it goes so we can work together on how to increase our Medicare reimbursement performance. Bonnie, in 45 days let's review what effect your strategy has had on our reimbursement percentage."

"Sure. And I'll jot down the specific steps I'm going to take and the objectives we need to achieve. I'll give you the outline tomorrow."

■ ■ ■

Understanding Financial Reports

Overview

Certified public accountants and other financial experts often treat ambulance managers paternalistically. They speak a language of mumbo jumbo that would make any normal person dizzy. To avoid this, managers must learn the language of these wizards. It's not easy, and like any foreign language, it takes time and practice to understand and speak this way. It also takes perseverance. On first reading, the information presented here may not be clear. If not, re-read it. You wouldn't expect to read French overnight, so don't be disappointed if this section requires several readings. Parlez-vous financial?

This section will help you understand important financial information about the service. Businesses throughout the world present financial pictures of their companies through financial statements—the common language used by those to whom the manager reports. This is true whether the service is public or private. These reports help us to understand what's going on inside the service. They reveal business trends and

(continued on next page)

(continued)

highlight opportunities and problems that would otherwise go unnoticed. If finance is difficult for you, choose someone on your board or in the community who will help you develop an understanding of the organization's finances. The reports reviewed in this section—*cash-flow summary, operating statement* and *balance sheet*—should be common to all ambulance services.

A manager uses the operating statement to answer questions about efficiency and profitability. Has the company met its financial goals? Have patient charges increased or decreased? Which expenses have increased or decreased and why? As administrator, ensure that assets and liabilities are proportionate, relative to each other and the service's activity. Be alert to the changing interrelationships between the operating statement and the balance sheet. And since a cash-flow summary is seldom included in financial reports, learn to derive the necessary cash-flow information from these two reports.

WHAT IS CASH FLOW?

Cash flow, simply put, is the actual inflow and outflow of cash. It's the heartbeat of any business. The cash-flow summary does *not* reveal profits or the service's financial condition. To measure profit, subtract all expenses from the total revenue. Obviously, money gained from borrowing, which is included in the cash-flow summary, cannot be included in the computation of profit. Similarly, disbursements for major equipment such as ambulance vehicles are long-term investments, and it is misleading to deduct their entire cost from a single year's revenue.

Cash flow doesn't represent all revenues and expense activities for the year. The cash coming in during the year doesn't represent the total year's ambulance revenues or sales activities. Since patients don't usually pay for ambulance services at the time of call, much revenue will be received later. Often forgotten by ambulance service managers is the spread of accounts receivable and its potentially disastrous effect on cash flow. This varies greatly, depending on those paying as well as the mix of patient accounts (for example, insurance companies, Medicare, Medicaid or self-pay) and on the collection practices of the service.

Likewise, cash disbursements don't measure total expenses for the year. There will be money paid out which will be tied up in inventory, there will be liabilities for the money the service owes to suppliers, as well as portions of interest payments and possible income-tax expenses. In other words, the money actually paid out by the company during a certain period will not necessarily match the bills the company accrued during the same period.

The actual financial condition of the ambulance service is measured by the size of its assets (inventory and accounts receivable) and liabilities (loans, bills and payables). This is not revealed in cash-

Figure 3.6 Sample Balance Sheet

CRISS CROSS AMBULANCE SERVICE
BALANCE SHEET
December 31

ASSETS	Current year	Prior year	LIABILITIES & FUND BALANCE	Current year	Prior year
CURRENT ASSETS:			CURRENT LIABILITIES:		
Cash on Hand	100	100	Accounts Payable	5,952	5,975
Cash in Bank	6,343	10,292	Payroll Taxes Payable	5,329	4,375
Accounts Receivable	152,334	112,879	Accrued Expenses	7,141	7,190
Accounts Receivable Ambulance District	467		Current Maturities of Long Term Debt	64,000	64,000
Less: Allowance for Uncoll. Accts	(94,669)	(34,153)	Deferred Income– Courier Service	4,866	
Inventories–Estimated	8,424	8,424			
Prepaid Expenses	9,906	4,972	TOTAL CURRENT LIAB.	87,228	81,540
TOTAL CURRENT ASSETS	82,906	102,514	Long Term Debt		
FIXED ASSETS			Notes Payable	112,404	112,288
			Less: Current Matur.	(64,000)	(64,000)
Leasehold Improvements	17,916	16,954			
Office Furniture and Fixtures	33,492	23,750	TOTAL LONG TERM DEBT	48,404	48,288
Medical Equipment	160,440	138,607	Fund Balance		
Vehicles	157,257	105,824	Balance Beginning of year	158,281	141,461
Less: Accumulated Depreciation	(140,722)	(75,906)	Excess of Revenues Over Expenses	17,316	40,454
TOTAL FIXED ASSETS	228,383	209,229	Total Balance	175,597	181,915
TOTAL ASSETS	311,289	311,743	TOTAL LIABILITIES AND FUND BALANCE	311,289	311,743

flow statements. The profit performance is given in the operating statement (also called profit and loss or income statement). The actual financial condition is presented on the balance sheet. Figure 3.6 gives an example of a balance sheet.

OPERATING STATEMENT

Figure 3.7, an operating statement, summarizes patient revenues and expenses for one year. The top line represents the total revenue for patient care and the bottom line is the net income after all expenses

Figure 3.7   Sample Operating Statement

CRISS CROSS AMBULANCE SERVICE
OPERATING STATEMENT
December 31

REVENUES	Actual	Budget	Prior Yr.	YTD Act	YTD Bud	Tot Bud
Patient Revenues	44,277	46,946	43,915	549,725	563,354	563,354
Allowances & Uncollectible Accts						
Allowances	11,416		3,729	78,912		
Provision for Bad Debts	11,069		10,978	129,948		
Total Allowances	22,485	14,084	14.707	208,860	169,010	169,010
Net Patient Revenues	21,792	32,862	29,208	340,865	394,344	394,344
Other Revenues						
Contributions	-		5,392	227,994		
Interest	108		132	1,368		
Courier Service	973		-	6,813		
Training	1,350		-	2,700		
Total Non-Operating Revenue	2,431	19,410	5,524	238,875	232,928	232,928
Total Revenue	24,223	52,272	34,732	579,740	627,272	627,272
EXPENSES						
Salaries--Administrative	3,442	3,432	5,261	42,023	41,192	41,192
Salaries--Production	24,534	24,892	19,721	290,312	298,714	298,714
Employee Benefits	4,391	5,033	3,086	55,446	60,396	60,396
Supplies	2,044	3,016	4,409	24,373	36,196	36,196
Insurance	526	855	527	6,311	10,262	10,262
Vehicle Maint. & Expense	1,820	2,568	2,787	18,931	30,826	30,826
Occupancy	1,953	1,746	1,607	22,227	20,952	20,952
Telephone	962	528	360	5,844	6,345	6,345
Postage	327	313	216	3,723	3,758	3,758
Depreciation	4,771	5,000	4,771	57,252	60,000	60,000
Interest	1,124	1,416	454	16,264	17,000	17,000
Other Expenses	2,405	2,219	1,195	19,718	26,631	26,631
Total Expenses	48,299	51,018	44,394	562,524	612,272	612,272
Excess Revenue (Expenses)	(24,076)	1,254	(9,662)	17,316	15,000	15,000

have been deducted. The income statement is read top to bottom, step by step. First, revenues are presented. Then expenses are deducted one by one until they've all been subtracted. In many businesses the "other revenues" are not included on the operating statement. But by including them, you'll have a more accurate picture of how your service is doing at a given moment.

The following accounting principles will help you determine if the revenues and expenses are being measured correctly.

Revenues. The total amount collected from ambulance services, or other patient services, during the year.

Operating expenses. Generally speaking, all expenses other than depreciation, interest and income tax.

Depreciation expense. That fraction of the original cost of all long-term assets, such as buildings, ambulances or large pieces of medical equipment, to be deducted from this year's revenue. It's the charge for using the assets during this period.

Interest expense. The total interest, and other financial charges, on debts for the year.

Income-tax expense. For private for-profit services, this will be the amount due to government on taxable income for the period, less any credits or deductions.

BALANCE SHEET

The balance sheet summarizes the assets and liabilities for the year or other operating period. The assets are divided into three groups.

Current assets. The current assets consist of cash-on-hand (in the bank), and other assets which could be readily converted into cash, such as certificates of deposit, inventory and accounts receivable.

Fixed assets. Ambulances, buildings, and equipment are examples of fixed assets. The cost is gradually deducted over the useful lifetime of the assets. This amount will be listed as depreciation, and the cumulative amount that has been deducted since acquisition is listed as accumulated depreciation.

Other assets. Other assets are those which are neither current nor fixed.

Liabilities are claims on, and sources of, assets. Money from loans and unpaid expenses increase a company's assets. By listing the liabilities, you can determine where the company's total assets came from.

There are interlocking relationships between the three types of statements. Net income (sometimes called excess revenue) or expenses is taken from the operating statement and is used as the starting point to compute cash outflow. The following paragraphs review some of the interrelating components.

Patient revenue—accounts receivable. When a patient is billed, the amount is entered into the patient-revenue account. At the end of the accounting period, the balance in the account is the sum total of all patient charges for the year–in this case, $549,725.

A certain portion of these patient charges, however, haven't been paid. Essentially, these services have been provided on credit. The total amount owed the service is listed in accounts receivable.

As you know, there are quick, regular and slow-paying customers. So, there will always be some charges that remain uncollected. As a rule, an ambulance service should keep its accounts receivable below, or less than, the equivalent of 90 days of average daily patient charges. This means that no more than 12 weeks of the service's yearly patient charges should remain uncollected. Naturally, the longer the period, the larger the accounts receivable. In the Criss Cross example, the service has about 101 days in accounts receivable.

Total Annual Patient Charges $549,725	÷	365 days	=	Average Daily Charges $1,506

Accounts Receivable $152,334	÷	Average Daily Charges $1,506	=	Number Of Days In Accounts Receivable 101 days

A shorter period means increased cash and decreased necessary borrowing. This eases cash-flow problems and saves interest on short-term loans.

Operating expenses—accounts payable. Operating expenses include all the expenses needed to operate a business—except depreciation. Rent, wages, payroll taxes, fringe benefits, office supplies, telephone, utilities, insurance and marketing are generally included.

Every operating-expense dollar, however, can't be considered a dollar actually disbursed; some operating expenses are recorded *before* they're paid. Examples of such expenses include utility bills, bills from lawyers, bills from suppliers and advertising bills. Therefore, at the end of the year some of these bills remain unpaid. This portion is listed in accounts payable.

Even though a bill or invoice for goods and services is immediately listed in accounts payable, this doesn't decrease cash. The recording of all bills is necessary in order to recognize the service's liabilities. In the Criss Cross example, the amount is the sum of accounts payable and payroll-taxes payable, or $11,281. This amount is equal to about seven days of the year's total expenses, which is within reasonable standards.

Operating expenses—prepaid expenses. These expenses, such as insurance premiums, are paid before they're recorded. They are initially listed in prepaid expenses, an asset account. During the year each month is charged its share of the total, for example insurance coverage. This amount is then taken out of prepaid expenses and recorded as operating expenses to be deducted from the revenue. Attempt to keep your total prepaid expenses to a minimum, because the money will be tied up and can increase cash-flow problems.

Fixed-asset depreciation expense. Fixed refers to assets with long and useful lives. For example, if an ambulance has a useful life of five years, one-fifth the total cost would be deducted each year.

As a fixed asset is depreciated, the amount in the fixed asset account doesn't decrease. Instead the accumulated depreciation is listed separately in the accumulated depreciation account. The portion of fixed assets not yet depreciated is usually listed as book value. Each year the book value decreases until it's eventually considerably less than the replacement costs of the fixed assets.

Interest expense. When a company borrows money, the liability is listed as notes payable because interest is paid on the money borrowed. Interest is reported as a separate cost—interest expense. The unpaid portion of interest at the end of the year is listed in accrued expenses.

Income-tax expense—income-tax payable. A portion of the estimated income tax is paid throughout the year. The remaining amount is listed in the income-tax payable account.

Net income—fund balance (retained earnings). Net income or excess revenue is the final profit after all expenses have been deducted from revenue. It increases the balance in the fund balance. Two things should be noted. First, patient revenue results in asset increases and expenses result in asset decreases or liability increases. Second, net income results from a combination of increases and decreases in several asset and liability accounts.

Net income doesn't mean money in the bank. In fact, cash can actually decrease from net income. The fund balance can also increase or decrease in response to net income.

The fund balance is *not* an asset. Instead, it helps determine how much equity is in the business. In a private company, this fund-balance amount is compared to the amount invested by the owners.

STATEMENTS OF SOURCES AND USES OF CASH

To figure net income, deduct your expenses from the revenue. Since revenues and expenses are generally recorded before and after cash flow, net income must be adjusted for changes in operating assets and changes in operating liabilities. Increases in assets use cash, while an increase in operating liabilities frees cash.

Increases in assets can be financed by increases in operating liabilities. Most of the money is generally raised through loans and other sources and sometimes from operation activites.

The net income and the *changes* in assets and liabilities determine where the cash came from and to what use it was put.

IMPACT OF GROWTH ON CASH FLOW

Growth is essential. Yet, unless there's an increase in patient revenues and expenses, with little or no increase in current assets, growth will penalize cash flow. If there's a 20 percent increase in business and patient revenues *as well as* expenses and assets, the cash available can actually drop. If this happens, the service may not be able to meet all of its financial obligations.

How much cash should be on hand? A valid question, indeed. The ambulance industry is unpredictable as well as labor intensive. Therefore, more ready cash is needed to meet unexpected emergencies. Sixty days of annual sales should provide an adequate cushion. Bankers, accountants and businessmen from other industries may feel a company should have three weeks or more of its annual sales revenue, or 9 percent of its total assets, available in cash, but this isn't a wide enough safety margin for the ambulance industry. If your service receives total subsidies once or twice a year, consider your safety margin so you don't run out of money before the next subsidy payment.

Cash-flow statements are often not included in financial reports, but sometimes a statement of changes in financial position may be. A cash-flow statement reports the sources and uses of *cash*. The statement of changes reports the sources and uses of *funds*. Funds are short-term working capital, and are computed by subtracting total current liabilities from total current assets.

FOOTNOTES TO FINANCIAL STATEMENTS

Footnotes are necessary for adequate disclosure in financial reports. There are two types. The first type of footnote covers major accounting principles such as depreciation methods or any accounting methods unique to that particular industry. The other type of footnote includes maturity dates, interest rates, collateral, other security provisions and any major lawsuits pending. There's still a good deal of management disagreement over how much the footnote should reveal. Footnote writing is often so unclear, awkward and overly technical that one suspects deliberate confusion to cover up poor business decisions.

FINANCIAL AUDITS

If you're audited by a CPA, he'll ask himself two questions. Is your company's accounting system performing reliably? Do all accounting decisions and methods comply with generally accepted accounting principles? If the auditor answers yes to both questions, a clean or unqualified opinion is given. If not, a qualified opinion is given. The qualified opinion means that, in general, the financial report is fair, but perhaps one of the company's accounting procedures doesn't comply with the generally accepted accounting principles, or the extent and manner of disclosure is not adequate.

Are audits required? That depends on the organization's structure. Some government services, as well as services with government contracts that use taxpayer's money, may be periodically required to undergo an audit. The governing body or a bank may require an audit before it will loan money. Unless the company stock is traded on a stock exchange or the company is trying to raise capital through securities, it's unlikely that a certified audit will be required. Even if an audit isn't required, it adds credibility to a company's financial statements.

If the cost of a full audit is too high, a service may request a review. A review is not an affirmative opinion, but a negative assurance. It says only that the CPA is not *aware* of any modifications needed to make the financial statements conform with generally accepted accounting principles.

IN SUMMARY. . .

As the pace quickens in the EMS industry, the successful manager will need more financial skills than ever before, yet these skills are some of the most difficult for an EMS manager to master. Why? Because the image of studiously pouring over figures like a banker or accountant is inconsistent with the image of making life-and-death decisions—the way most EMS managers see themselves.

Although financial statements may seem dry and boring, they clearly reveal the organization's financial health. By understanding what the statements are saying, you'll be able to make better managerial decisions which will in turn affect the well-being of the service. In addition, once you master the financial lingo, you'll be able to communicate with bankers, accountants, board members and councilmen.

C A S E   S T U D Y   # 6

Cash Flow

John, executive director of Ambassador Ambulance Service, readies himself for an 8:30 meeting with his operations manager, Tom. Tom is to present the financial pro formas for the impending takeover of Flintstone County. Flintstone County residents have been unhappy for a number of years with their previous ambulance service and have recently requested that Ambassador add their county to its service area.

The board of directors supported the idea in principle but wanted a presentation on the financial impact of such a decision.

Tom's been working on the financial presentation for the last four weeks. He had asked John if he could prepare the pro formas on his own, and John had agreed.

And so, for the next thirty minutes, Tom presents his work. It's comprehensive and clear. He has prepared a two-page executive summary in which he reviews the project and its financial impact. The next 20 pages provide justification, explanation, budget, and operating statements for the first year's operation.

John checks off his list of questions. Yes, the capital expenditures are appropriate. Tom's amortized the purchases over correct life cycles and has even included the repayment of principle and interest. Salaries are consistent with proposed unit hours and the unit-hour projections provide proper use ratios.

"Tom, the expense side looks good. Let's look a little closer at the revenues. I see that your operating statement for the first year shows an excess of revenue. That's good, but frankly better than I would have expected. How did you calculate the revenues?"

"Well, I spent a lot of time discussing this with Bonnie. Charges and Medicare profiles of the current provider are identical with ours. Since our charges are public information, they've always matched their charges with ours. Neither of us could come up with a reason why collections should be any different. The demographics, such as age and income, are similar. Transport distance shouldn't vary much from our history. But, to be safe, we estimated collection in the new area at 5 percent lower than our 70 percent."

"Okay, that sounds good. But, something's missing. What about start-up operating capital?"

"I thought about that. Bonnie assured me that our office can dispense insurance claims and bills the day after we begin service. With a 65 percent collection rate, we should be fine."

"Well, Tom, I think we've found the missing link. Let's talk this through," John says, "and figure out what money will be coming in. We don't get the current operator's accounts, so we don't receive payments for services done before we start. Don't we generally collect about 15 percent of the charges within 30 days of the date of service?

Which, of course, doesn't mean we'll collect 15 percent of the first month's charges by the end of the month. It just means that 30 days after the first day, we can predict collection of 15 percent of that day's charges. So, by the end of the second month, we'll have collected 15 percent of the first month's charges plus a much smaller percentage from the second month's charges. Tom, you know it's not easy to accurately predict the incoming cash from a new operation, so the best we can do is use past information to get an approximation.

"Tom, your prepared history shows 15 percent of the charges are collected within 30 days. An additional 30 percent is collected in the 30- to 60-day period. Twelve and a half percent more is collected from 60 to 90 days from the date of service. Seven and a half percent from 90 to 120 days and the final 5 percent is squeezed out of accounts over 120 days. Since you're predicting 5 percent less in collections from the new area, let's subtract 1 percent from each of the collection periods.

"That'll give us . . .

0–30 days	14.0%
30–60 days	29.0%
60–90 days	11.5%
90–120 days	6.5%
120–150 days	4.0%
for a total collection of	65.0%.

"That makes sense," says Tom, "but it's confusing."

"Okay, Tom, let's see if we can create a graph that illustrates what I'm talking about. If our monthly charges average $50,000 for Flintstone County, let's see what the first month's charges will generate in receipts and when."

John and Tom huddle around the micro-computer and boot up the spreadsheet program. They enter the numbers and calculate the percentage of the first month's charges and predict when the money will flow into the organization.

"Let's look at the graph," says John after the calculations and numbers have been entered. "Neglecting the minimal amount that might come in in the first month, we see that at the end of the second month we'll have received $7,000 from the first month's charges. By the end of the third month, an additional $14,500 should have come in from the first month's charges. After that, it starts to decline—an additional $5,750 by the end of the fourth month, $3,250 by the end of the fifth and $2,000 by the end of the sixth month."

"I think I understand," says Tom, "but aren't these figures only the receipts generated from the first month's billings? What about the billings for the second and following months?"

"Right," says John. "And to do that we'll add to our graph. If we consider the same collections and the same average charges for the rest of the year, we'll get a more complete graphic picture of the first year's receipts."

John enters more data for revenue from additional months and prints out the chart.

"John, I agree. But our collection rate doesn't peak until after the sixth month of operation."

"That's right, Tom. It takes a long time for collections to achieve maximum effectiveness. As you can see by the chart, significant receipts aren't received until after the third month of operation. That's why we have to be careful about cash flow. There won't be enough cash coming into the organization to fund operations until after five months. We'll have to be able to cover this negative cash-flow period when expenses are more than receipts."

"OK, we've projected that expenses will average $30,000 per month for the Flintstone operation." Tom draws a line across the graph at the $30,000 level. "So, if I add up the differences between the expenses and the receipts for the first five months, we'll have an idea of how much available cash we'll need. Then, if I add start-up expenses, such as uniforms, non-capital equipment, supplies, rent and so on, we'll know the total start-up capital required. But wait! This means the total cash received won't equal the total cash going out for the first year. We'll lose money!"

"You're probably right," John says, "but let's do the same analysis for the second and third years. If we can break even by the end of the third year, I'm sure the board will approve. Generally, a new business takes two or three years before it starts to break even."

John and Tom return to work on the computer satisfied that the presentation will be accurate, complete, and ready for the board's review.

■   ■   ■

The Procurement Process

Overview

Purchasing! We all like to buy things. Whether personal or for the service, most of us get a thrill out of buying. This is one reason why procurement policies need to be well defined.

Procurement means purchasing goods and services for use by the organization. The following policies and procedures will help you ensure judicious purchasing.

Limit the number of people authorized to buy things. Make sure you get what you need and need what you get. Get the best possible price. Make sure the service can afford it. Ensure that the purchase will benefit the organization. Make sure you get what you pay for. And finally, keep track of all expenditures for goods and services.

WHO SHOULD PURCHASE

Most services don't have a large enough staff to employ a full-time purchasing agent, so the responsibility for purchasing is usually added work for the manager or other management personnel. The responsibility for approving a purchase generally should be handled by one person in the organization.

Some systems either require the board treasurer's approval or full board's approval for *all* purchases. This system is time consuming and should be altered. After all, what are they paying the manager for? Most governing bodies reserve the right to approve large purchases— for example, anything which costs more than $1,000. For your protection as well as the governing body's information, set a lower limit of $500 for approval of non-budgeted items. It's also a good idea for the EMS administrator to have the authority to sign checks with a single signature up to a specified limit like $1,000. Anything over that amount would require that checks be co-signed by a board officer or owner. This process streamlines day-to-day activities by saving valuable time. It also gives you the additional protection to ensure this right isn't abused.

As manager, you may want to delegate some of your purchasing authority as the board has done to you. For example, you might allow the operations' manager or a specifically designated field employee to purchase necessary replacement supplies or maintenance items up to a specified limit, say $150. The office manager might be allowed purchasing authority for office supplies up to a $50 limit. The purchase limit will vary depending on the size of your organization and your assessment of each supervisor. Strictly limit to one or two trusted people the authority to buy without prior approval. These entrusted few will then take their responsibilities seriously.

Every item purchased, even those ordered through your delegated authority, should be documented on a purchase request form.

SPECIFICATIONS

A good procurement process ensures you get exactly what you need. The business of prehospital health care requires a large amount of specialized equipment and supplies. Part of the manager's job is to determine exactly which items are needed. Part of this process is facilitated by creating detailed specifications for each purchase. The specifications for a particular item may be as simple as sterile 4″ × 4″ gauze dressings in packages of two or as complex as a 30-page document detailing the many requirements for a new Type II ambulance.

Good specifications are a key to making sure you get what you need and want. Plus, once you've detailed your specifications, you can use them over again making minor changes to reflect any new requirements or errors in the first set of specs. This provides uniformity in the equipment and also reduces retraining the team for entirely new designs on similar equipment. As you prepare specifications, don't forget to seek input from those who will use the new items. They're the ones who know what's needed and what to avoid. The specifications must be precise so the vendor knows what's required and can respond accordingly to variances between the company's equipment and specifications. They should be written generically so you can receive the best price from a variety of vendors.

PRICE CONSIDERATIONS

Bids. Detailed specifications allow you to request bids from various suppliers. Send the specifications with a letter containing information about the number of items needed, the date by which the bids need to be returned, when the purchase decision will be made and the name and number of the person to contact if there are any questions. Any other pertinent information regarding the procurement should be included. Request any specifications that can't be met by the vendor or substitutes to be documented. Lengthy specifications should provide a yes or no box beside each specified item so that the vendor can mark whether or not his product meets that requirement. A complete and signed copy of the specification sheet should be included in all bids.

After the bids have been received, they must be carefully examined to make sure that each of the vendor's products complies with the specifications and to determine which vendor offers the best price. Many governmental entities must take the lowest bid that meets the specifications. If your service isn't limited by such requirements, you have the advantage of haggling. Contact the top few vendors to see if an even better deal can be negotiated. It never hurts to try.

Price shopping. For smaller routine items, the bidding is too time consuming and expensive. The same benefits can be enjoyed by price shopping. If you were going to buy a TV set for your home, you'd probably check around for the best price. The same effort will benefit your organization. Either telephone or personally visit to check the different prices from various suppliers. You'll realize significant savings. The request-for-purchase form, when used for telephone or letterhead bids, should be designed so that prices from at least three separate vendors can be listed.

Negotiations. The nature of our business can help the manager get the best deal. We help people. Many businessmen are willing to give ambulance services a special discount because of our good-guy image. But these discounts won't seek *you* out. Instead, you have to personally develop the civic mindedness of businessmen to secure pricing advantages.

Negotiations based on the volume of goods or services you purchase is another effective technique. For example, if your service doesn't have an in-house mechanic, you can negotiate saying you'll need a sizable amount of mechanical services. It there are enough qualified suppliers to bid on the mechanical services, or if you've identified the best source to meet your needs, then negotiation is called for. It's often possible to negotiate a lower hourly rate if you're willing to devote some personal time and effort to the supplier.

Negotiating can also be called haggling. You and your staff should always try for a better price. It never hurts to ask, and the savings can be enormous.

Volume buying. You already know that if you buy large quantities it's often possible to get a better unit price. Buying 55 gallons of bulk oil or antifreeze can save money over purchasing cans or cases. Buying a case of glass cleaner can be significantly cheaper than purchasing individual bottles. A word to the wise—don't overdo it. One service we know bought 20 cases of normal saline-injection solution on sale. They were using about one IV of normal saline per month. At the end of the year they had 19 cases of outdated IV solutions. They didn't save any money.

It's not a good idea to buy *everything* in large quantities, but you might consider buying frequently used items that won't spoil or become outdated in bulk quantities. You tie up a great deal of money in inventory if you don't use caution in your buying habits.

Another type of volume buying is group purchasing. Hospitals often band together to buy large quantities of a particular item at low unit cost. They then divide the products among themselves. They've used the advantage of bulk purchasing but don't have to tie up too much of their resources in inventory. Ambulance services across the country have also formed organizations to accomplish the same goal. It's well worth exploring the possibility of joining or forming such an association.

It might be possible for your service to purchase some of its supplies directly from regional hospitals. They often get the best price and might be willing to pass some of their savings on to your service.

Government services may be able to take advantage of their status in the buyer's market. For example, a tire franchise had a state contract to supply state vehicles with tires. The tire-store manager legally supplied the municipal service with tires at a state rate. The service purchased its tires at half price, 25 percent lower than what a high-volume commercial company was able to negotiate.

Remember, if your service is governmental or non-profit, it's tax exempt. You don't pay sales taxes—even on small purchases.

Many vendors award discounts on the prompt payment of invoices. Don't miss this opportunity. Either pay these invoices first and collect the discounts, or don't pay the bill until it's due. Keep the service's money earning interest as long as possible.

Is the item needed? Before any manager approves a purchase request, it's necessary to ensure the item is really needed. Will the purchase of this item enable employees to perform their jobs better? Will it provide better patient care? Will it help the office function more efficiently? Will it be used? These and other questions need to be answered to ensure that the purchase of the item is appropriate and not just a Christmas wish. It must provide a tangible benefit to justify the expense.

Can the service afford it? Has the expense been budgeted and can the service afford the purchase at this time? If the expense doesn't fit into your budget, look closer. The budget was created and approved to provide guidelines for purchases. Non-budgeted items, as a rule, shouldn't be purchased unless they are absolutely essential. *If you don't follow your own budget, who will?*

Even something that's budgeted may not be affordable. If income hasn't matched projections, or if expenses have been running over, the new purchase may have to wait until cash flow improves. It's the manager's responsibility to weigh all of these points before approving a purchase.

Get what you pay for. After an item is ordered, make sure that you get what you ordered. When it's delivered, a receiving report should be completed, noting what has been received and what was possibly back ordered. The receiving report may be a separate form or a packing slip requiring the signature of the person receiving the shipment. Make sure everything is undamaged and operable. Any shortcomings should be noted and the vendor contacted to affect corrections prior to payment. The packing slip, receiving report and request for purchase forms should all be reviewed before payment is made to the vendor. This assures that you get what you pay for and helps avoid double payments.

Keeping track. This whole system is designed to save money and keep track of each purchase expenditure. The next section describes a specific procurement plan which includes many of the points already discussed. It may seem complex, but it's not as difficult as it appears. The system is necessary to avoid costly errors and misunderstandings.

STEPS FOR AN EFFECTIVE PURCHASING SYSTEM

Figure 3.8 demonstrates an effective purchasing plan. We'll now outline each step in enough detail for you to create your own system.

Step 1. Someone decides that the service needs to buy something. This idea generally comes from the operations' personnel, office staff or administration including the board. At this time a purchase-request form (PRF) is filled out. The purchase-request form should include more than one item. Item descriptions, reasons for requesting each purchase and the manufacturer's identification number should be filled in. The person requesting the purchase signs and dates the form and it's then routed to the operations' or office manager.

Step 2. The operations' or office manager completes the vendor and pricing information. Three different vendors should be listed with their catalog numbers and individual item descriptions. Get prices from each supplier and document them. Any comments, special requests or vendor recommendations should be included before the manager signs his or her approval to the request. The PRF then goes to the director. (If it exceeds the delegated amount, the manager is allowed to singularly purchase.)

Step 3. The director then reviews the request. If the request is for a large amount or if it's for a new piece of equipment that will be frequently purchased, the administrator may decide to initiate a formal bid process or request the development of detailed specifications. If so, the PRF would be returned to the manager with instructions.

If a formal process isn't needed, then the director asks these questions. Is the item(s) needed? Is it accounted for in the budget? To which account should it be charged? Finally, can the service afford the item at this time? Let's say the director decides to purchase. He'll indicate as such on the PRF, saying whether or not it's budgeted, what account should be charged and the vendor selected. Then the PRF

Figure 3.8   Purchasing-System Diagram

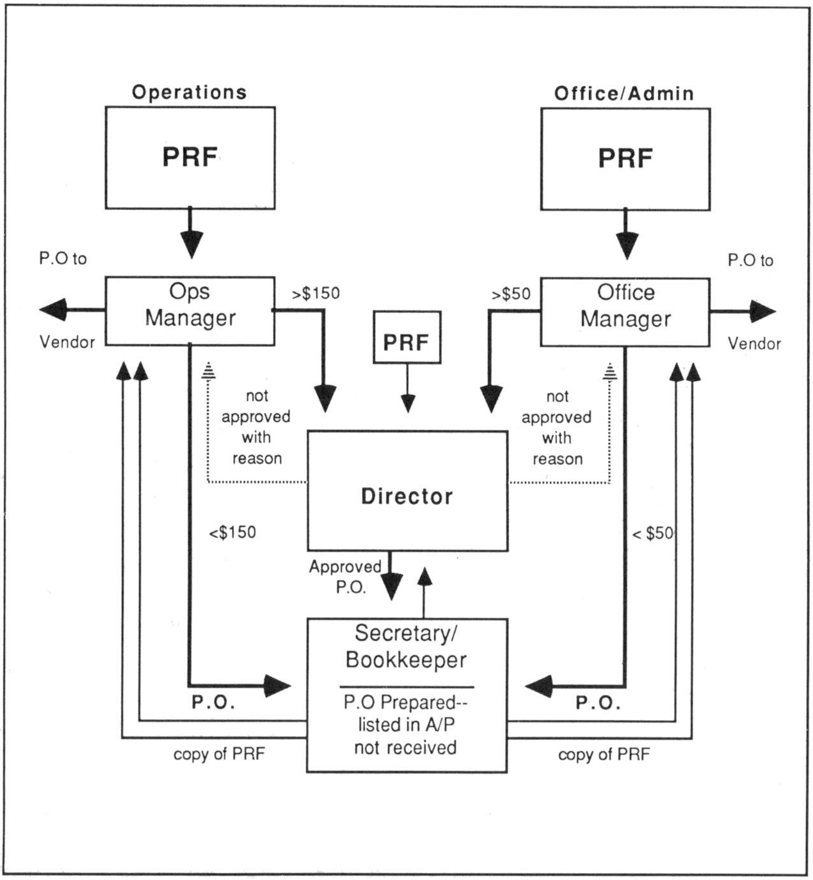

is signed, dated and passed to the secretary or bookkeeper for action.

Step 4. The secretary or bookkeeper uses the PRF to create a purchase order (PO). Purchase orders are consecutively numbered, like checks in a checkbook. One copy is sent to the vendor to place the order. The other is retained for records. The secretary will enter the PO number on the PRF and return the PRF and PO to the operations' or office manager. This person also documents the order and places the copy of the PO in a holding file that lists the items not yet received. This enables the bookkeeper to keep track of committed funds for future invoices.

Step 5. The operations' or office manager then sends the PO to the vendor and keeps the PRF until receiving the material. It may work better for your service to have the secretary mail the PO and keep the PRF until the shipment arrives.

This process, or something like it, should be the routine for procuring supplies and equipment. It sounds complicated, but in actual practice it streamlines the purchasing process while keeping close control over the entire system. Variations will occur if the PRF originates from the director. The director can be bypassed if he or she has delegated limited purchasing authority to the managers.

RECEIVING

Many organizations have trouble keeping track of newly received material. New items have a way of getting on ambulances without anyone knowing how or when they got there. It's important to develop a procedure to avoid this. The receiving diagram in Figure 3.9 shows how to keep this from happening. The various steps follow.

Step 1. As supplies and materials are received, they are checked by whomever ordered them. A receiving report is completed, any missing or damaged items noted and the vendor contacted immediately. The items received and back ordered are listed on the receiving report. If the shipment is complete, the packing slip, PRF and receiving report are forwarded to the secretary or bookkeeper for processing. If the order isn't complete, a *copy* of the PRF is attached to the packing slip and the receiving report marked incomplete and then forwarded to the secretary or bookkeeper.

Step 2. The secretary or bookkeeper attaches these forms to the copy of the PO in the old holding file (for purchases which have been ordered but not received), and moves them to another holding file (for purchases which have been received but are awaiting invoices).

Step 3. When the invoice arrives from the vendor, attach the holding-file information to the invoice and note any early-payment discounts. This information is then moved to the accounts-payable file which keeps track of all purchases.

Step 4. As the manager, review the accounts-payable file once or twice a month to determine payment. Review each purchase and bill to ensure the proper account number is on each PO and statement and to determine which vendors need paying.

Figure 3.9   Receiving-System Diagram

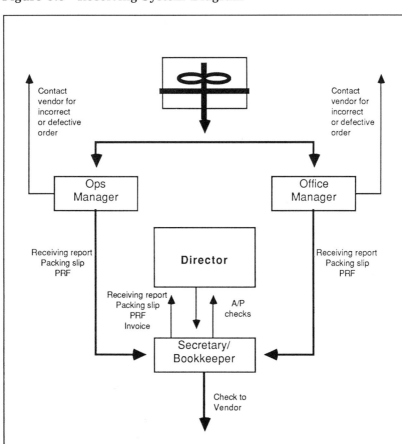

Step 5. Transfer bills to be paid to the bookkeeper who'll prepare the checks for the manager's signature and attach them to any information included about each purchase and account.

Step 6. Review the information, verify the accuracy of each check and its account, sign the checks and return them to the bookkeeper who will post and mail them.

This system works because every purchase is reviewed as it crosses the desks of both the bookkeeper and the director. The system's built-in checks and balances prevents errors and double payments. In a large service, some of the responsibilities may be passed to other specialized managers, and in a smaller service some of the duties will be combined. But the basic procedure should stand.

One final hint—*never purchase items with cash.* Of course there are always exceptions. It would be ridiculous to write a $.02 check for postage due. Make petty cash available for *small* purchases, but even then, document everything to the penny. The use of checks forces documentation and makes it easier to keep track of expenditures, whereas the handling of cash always involves some risk.

A procurement system provides control and makes keeping track of expenditures easier. And it has the added advantage of documenting good purchasing practices.

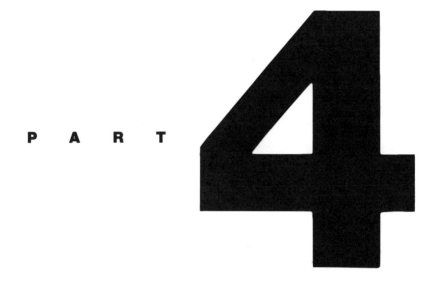

Calling the Plays—
Operational Matters

Quality
Assurance

Overview

The goal of an EMS system or ambulance service is to provide patients with the best possible care at a reasonable cost. In order to do this, the service delivering that care must be organized. There are two important qualities which enable the organization to deliver appropriate care. First, the staff must be capable and motivated to offer their best efforts for the patients. The importance of personnel selection can't be overstressed. In order for patients to receive quality care, the service's caregivers must be competent, well-trained, and have the experience necessary to make difficult decisions and take lifesaving actions in stressful, adverse situations.

Second, the system must be *designed* for excellence. Even the most competent team members can't deliver high-quality care in poorly designed and managed ambulance services. Of course, a well-designed service structure, by itself, won't deliver good patient care. The system's structure must be built to facilitate patient care. Combined with high-quality prehospital medical personnel must be a framework that is

(continued on next page)

(continued)

medically and operationally sound to ensure success. Who benefits from a well-designed system? *Everyone!* Patients, taxpayers, employees and management personnel.

This section explores some of the fundamental building blocks necessary to construct a solid system. First, determine if the system is functioning as you'd like it to. To measure this objectively, there must be a quality-assurance process.

Paramedics and EMTs are essentially extensions of the system's physician advisor or other responsible physician. This relationship between physician and the prehospital medical person is often ignored. Technicians in the ambulance industry have been trained to use a specific set of skills. These skills are medically sound procedures which, prior to the evolution of prehospital emergency medical services, were performed in hospitals by nurses and doctors. Today, these procedures are done in the field resulting in immediate life-saving care.

Many street medics haven't looked closely enough at their relationship with physicians and nurses to fully understand the hierarchy. This is particularly true with paramedic personnel. Paramedics can function only because legislation in their state enables them to perform certain procedures under the direction of a physician. They are the eyes, ears and hands of the emergency-room doctor. They operate under that doctor's license as his extension or surrogate. The physician is legally responsible for the paramedic's actions. That legal liability is a major financial and ethical concern for the physician and the base hospital. Fortunately for patients, most physicians are willing to take on this added responsibility in order to provide immediate medical assistance.

Ambulance services, paramedics, EMTs, hospitals and physicians must establish guidelines and policies to reduce that potential liability between physicians and paramedics and to ensure high-quality medical care is given to *all* patients. The links in this chain are a medical-control point, the service's medical director, run-report documentation and call review. First, we'll discuss medical control.

MEDICAL CONTROL

Medical control is the link which provides patient-care instructions and direct medical supervision of field personnel. Ideally, there should be direct communication between the physician and the paramedic in the field. This direct linkage allows the physician to get a clear word picture of the patient's condition and circumstance. With additional exchange of information, the physician can give proper directions, and the paramedic will be more comfortable with the procedures he must perform.

A designated registered nurse sometimes assists the doctor in giving the field personnel directions. If designated RNs are used, it's important that they receive the necessary training and support to help them act in crisis situations.

Some states provide for the operation of paramedical personnel on standing orders either for specific overall-treatment guidelines or for special circumstances. There are clearly written procedures which outline techniques that can be used prior to contacting medical control or without any medical control communication. Special-circumstance exceptions provide the paramedic with specific steps to take when radio communications fail. In California, for example, standing orders are well-accepted although they vary greatly from county to county.

There are many pitfalls with standing orders. It's wise for a service to limit the use of standing orders when possible. Local physicians must be involved in their development and agree to their use. Careful documentation of the circumstances and use of standing orders is mandatory. The legal implications of the use of standing orders is also of concern. Some states expressly forbid their use, some states specifically legislate or regulate their use and some states have the special-circumstance provision for standing-order use. If your service is considering the use of standing orders, be sure to explore the legal restrictions and attitudes of those doctors who are ultimately responsible.

A functional medical-control plan will contain the following:

1. Direct radio communications with a physician experienced in emergency-medical care and familiar with local EMS protocols and operations.
2. Critical-care nurses who are trained in local EMS protocols and

are familiar with local EMS operations and who can stand in for the control physician if necessary.

3. Identification of medical facilities and establishment of transport protocols for the delivery of patients based on severity and type of injury or illness or proximity to the scene.

4. A uniform and complete set of medical protocols approved by the regulatory agency.

5. Paramedics and other field personnel, known to the medical-control physicians, who know the protocols and operations of the system.

6. A method to evaluate patient care and functioning of the system, with appropriate feedback to the operations personnel, both in the hospital and in the EMS service.

7. Backup systems, in the case of radio failure, emergency-department overload, disasters and other unforeseen problems.

In summary, effective medical control doesn't just mean talking to a doctor at the other end of a telephone or radio. The support and design of your system must communicate that paramedical personnel are extensions of the physician, and must be held accountable as such.

THE ROLE OF THE MEDICAL DIRECTOR

Another important link that strengthens the chain of excellent medical care is the service's medical director. His role in determining both the quality of patient care and the competency of the field personnel shouldn't be overlooked.

The role played by many medical directors is that of a figurehead to simply "meet the regulatory agency's requirements." That is *not* the purpose of the medical director. It's a waste for the service, the physician and the community if the medical director is not fully involved. The medical director lends expertise to both the system's operation and the patient's treatment. The medical director reviews and makes suggestions for medical protocols as well as keeps the service current as new technologies and treatments evolve. Reviewing patient outcomes and treatments in the field is under the control of the medical director. He verifies the training level of the field personnel, assists in their continuing education and routinely challenges personnel to demonstrate their practical skills. New medical equipment, medications and technologies should be studied by the medical director prior to their acquisition or use. In an enhanced role, the medical director provides liaison with the physicians in the community and hospital facilities, serves as a leader in garnering public support through public relations efforts, and is a sounding board for the service's manager.

A medical director is necessary for both ALS and BLS services. He should be an integral member of the team, should be well-known to the EMTs, paramedics and other staff and should know the operations of the service.

TRAINING AND CONTINUING EDUCATION

The training program used by an EMS system can be a key component of the service's quality-assurance program. Most states have adopted federal minimum standards for both EMT and paramedic training. Therefore, this section will concentrate on continuing education and management training opportunities— difficult areas for services.

Continuing medical education is vitally important to every ambulance service's operation. It assures excellent patient care. Too often, people complete their original training and become licensed without realizing their personal responsibility lies in keeping up with the fast-paced changes in this dynamic field. EMT and paramedic training is like buying a car. The initial investment is but a small part of the total amount spent over the life of the vehicle when one considers gas, tires, insurance, etc. Continuing education supports the EMTs' and paramedics' original investment in the training.

Some people argue that continuing education is not important. "I have a photographic memory. What I learned two years ago is so firmly embedded in my mind that I remember it completely." Or "The runs I make each day keep me completely qualified." These comments were among those made by a group of professionals. Humbug! Would you want them caring for your loved one?

Continuing education can actually be divided into two parts. The first part is refresher training. This involves review of the original training material to refresh the medic's knowledge. The second part adds new material to his original body of knowledge.

Opportunities for continuing education are limitless. Joint-training sessions with police, fire and other emergency officials can be arranged and will help improve on-scene relationships. Local physicians are often willing to donate their time for regular lectures. General management training opportunities for staff members are also available in most communities.

DOCUMENTATION

"If it isn't written down, it hasn't been done." This statement is central to documenting contact with patients. If you talk to an attorney—especially one who specializes in medical malpractice—you realize the importance of accurate and complete documentation. Sloppy and incomplete reports are a plaintiff attorney's delight. To avoid potential legal problems as well as embarrassment, review call-documentation procedures carefully.

There are a number of standardized formats for documenting a patient encounter. The format you select is not important, as long as it includes necessary and accurate information—neatly documented. As you evaluate your service's documentation procedures, look for these things.

Completeness. Obtain all relevant patient information—name, address, telephone number. Pay special attention to documenting the time and treatment procedures. How was the patient found? Where was he found? What environmental clues were there? Who else was there? Was there anything suspicious? What treatment was done prior to the ambulance's arrival? Were the patient's history and exams completely documented? Was treatment documented? (Remember— "If it isn't written, it wasn't. . . .")

Accuracy. The information must be accurate, and in many cases provable. Do not enhance the trip report. Not all patient encounters go well. Even so, the information must be reliable. Special emphasis must be placed on response time, specific treatment and delivery to the medical facility. It's a good idea for these times to be provable as well. Tape dispatch communications and log calls.

Neatness. This may seem trivial, but it's actually very important. The appearance of the report will reflect on the competence and professionalism of the service and its personnel. Imagine if you were to make a decision based on an incomplete and sloppy report! What would your first opinion of the author be? Many times, jurors make generous financial judgments based on their opinions of the opposing parties.

Observations, not judgments. Opinions of field personnel don't belong on a patient report. Observations, symptoms and actions should be described, but judgments and diagnosis should be avoided. Judgments such as "he was drunk" are inappropriate. They are *not* provable and will be embarrassing when brought out in court.

A patient's report is a confidential legal document and should be treated as such. Many hospitals append a copy of the run report to the patient's chart, where it's read by the emergency physicians, staff physicians, nurses, medical-records personnel and others. Every time it's read, the reader will form an opinion regarding the ambulance service. Let's make sure that the opinion is favorable. A sample run report is included as Appendix I.

The run report will also be an important tool to help service personnel and medical physicians review patient treatment for appropriateness and conformity to medical protocols. Establish a system to periodically review patient care. At this time, the EMTs, paramedics and physicians can discuss patient outcomes and determine if any improvement can be made in the prehospital care. These sessions shouldn't punish, to be called only when there has been a complaint. Instead, they should be routine. The purpose is not to catch somebody doing something wrong. The purpose is to identify the procedures and personnel *actions* which may need changing or improving. These sessions also allow for feedback to personnel about situations they handled well. They're a valuable tool for training as well as uncovering problems.

Field personnel should also be able to initiate review of a particular run. This is also true for the patient, family, emergency physicians, service administration, attending physicians, nursing personnel or any other person with *direct* knowledge of the assignment. The session should be open to any of the medical personnel and their participation encouraged. The sports analogy works well here. Call review is like a football team's Monday-morning sessions with the coach to review films of Sunday's game. Team spirit abounds. An objective attitude prevails. They ask, "How can we change the play or the way the team members run the play in order to win the game?"

The medical director should chair these meetings and the results recorded for those field personnel who can't attend. Most reviews of ambulance runs can be handled informally. Occasionally, a serious mistake or deliberate action made on a run may result in a more formal patient audit and definitive action toward an employee, protocol or medical facility.

Using client-feedback cards is another way in which a service can monitor quality. The pre-addressed card is sent to the patient before or with his first invoice. This has proven effective in determining client satisfaction at a reasonable cost. The card also provides services with impressive statistics for presentation. For example, "Of the 500 respondents, 96 percent indicated the service was excellent."

Having *systems* in place that monitor clinical care and customer satisfaction gives the EMS manager the tools to help the team focus on what's important. Quality-assurance systems provide vital information to help managers detect early in the game when things are not going as planned and what future plays may be more effective. The key point here bears repeating: all forms of retrospective incident review should be handled from a positive approach that builds team spirit and performance rather than from a critical, fault-finding perspective. If EMS coaches follow the prescription of 10 parts praise for every one part of criticism, their team will outperform their wildest expectations.

HANDLING COMPLAINTS

If you use the procedures outlined above, you'll eliminate many complaints about service. When a complaint does come in by phone, mail or in person, it should be handled in a professional way that doesn't give staff members the feeling of being interrogated. In fact, a good idea is not to call it a complaint procedure but rather a service inquiry.

Service inquiries are recorded in a central log kept by the manager or other management official. Depending on the seriousness of the allegation or problem, it may be handled by discussing the situation informally with the employee. More serious problems should be put in writing by all parties involved. Regardless of how it's handled with employees, a brief summary of the findings should be placed in the file, a disposition noted and a brief note sent or telephone call made to the original inquiring party. Most inquiries are resolved within 24 to 48 hours and the findings reported to the party immediately.

THE SERVICE MANUAL

One way the EMS manager distributes information to the team is by preparing a comprehensive set of guidelines and policies in the form of a service manual. Not only should specific procedures and policies be included, but statements about the history, philosophy and goals of the organization incorporated. The service manual defines the foundation of an EMS system's structure. It's the vital link in the chain for quality patient care. The procedures and function of the service are written down for all to see and to learn proper organizational procedures. The importance of a service manual can't be overstressed. If members of an organization aren't clear about their responsibilities, compliance can't be expected—and won't occur.

A good manual prevents various conflicts arising from unclear management directives. It reduces inaction by employees who are unclear about what's expected of them. The manual shouldn't be fixed in stone, however, but periodically updated when changing times require another approach and flexible enough to allow creative and innovative input from the EMS team. The policies should be dated and reviewed frequently by both management and staff with productive changes discussed and entered.

The manual provides an orientation for new employees to the organization philosophy, goals and performance expectations. Even personnel who have been with the organization for a long time will benefit from refresher training on the goals and policies in the manual. *Do not expect top performance unless you have clearly informed your personnel about their responsibilities.*

The manual improves interdepartmental communication. For example, field personnel will better understand the work being done in the billing department and vice versa. It will also help to standardize the quality of work from employees. It eliminates confusion by giving specific instructions. It facilitates the process of on-the-job training. The manual provides an effective way of maintaining current procedures by keeping team members aware of new equipment and accepted procedures. The manual also saves money by preventing duplication of functions and reducing errors caused by confusion. By including the organization's philosophies and goals, the manual increases confidence in the administration. It aids in the employee-appraisal process by providing guidelines from which to compare the employee's performance. It promotes teamwork within the organization. The manual assures compliance with legal requirements and legally protects the organization regarding personnel policies and care standards. The ambulance service's manual is useful in many other ways and is an integral part of quality assurance.

Now that the importance of a comprehensive and accurate manual has been outlined, does your service's manual stack up? Development of a manual is a complex task. If your manual isn't up to par, or if you don't have one, create one. The first step is to make an outline of the material you want included. The manual will open with a title page, followed by a letter from the director welcoming the employees. The table of contents is next. It should outline the major topics and subtopics in order of their appearance. A preface, written by the author of the manual, explains its purpose and how to use it. An introduction could be included to elaborate on its structure or content. Discuss your service's history. It interests new employees, and provides them with a perspective on the background, stability and future of the organization.

The core of the manual includes specific policies, procedures, guidelines and informational material.

The important parts of the manual, then, are:

1. *Introductory material.* The history, philosophy, organizational structure of the service and how to use the manual.

2. *Operations.* The policies and procedures for day-to-day operations as well as special circumstances. Information about on-scene command, communications, ambulance accidents, facility maintenance and description, maintenance of vehicles and equipment and a host of other material.

3. *Personnel policies.* The organization's policies and procedures regarding personnel. Job descriptions, probation, hiring, disciplinary actions, dress codes, performance appraisals, payroll and benefits are defined in this section.

4. *Patient-care policies.* The complete medical protocols and patient-encounter guidelines make up this all-important part of the manual.

As you write the manual, remember the difference between policies and procedures. *Policies* are explicit statements of organizational rules. They are not created haphazardly but are carefully designed to enhance job performance and patient care. They may be general or specific. General policies provide a *guide* for team members, whereas specific policies necessitate exact compliance. "No smoking in the ambulance" is an example of a specific policy. *Procedures*, on the other hand, are specific step-by-step descriptions of actions used to support a policy.

For example, a policy might state that the crew chief is responsible for patient care at the scene and en route to the patient's destination. The crew chief must ensure that the vehicle is at all times mechanically sound and clean. He or she verifies that all patient and run documentation is complete and accurate. This simplified policy for the crew chief is then supported by a number of procedures.

The procedures might include complete medical protocols, vehicle checklist and maintenance procedures, procedures for completing the run report, procedures for obtaining and documenting patient-billing information, vehicle cleaning and decontaminating procedures and communications' procedures.

Following are things to remember when creating policies and procedures. They shouldn't be arbitrary. Aim them toward the overall mission of the organization. It's unfortunate that many services fall into the trap of trying to dictate every step of an employee's action. Too many rules make for unhappy and confused team members. The policies must be carefully thought out, and each one must be valid and necessary. Authentic sources of information should be used for policy development and the policies can't conflict with legal or ethical imperatives. The policies should be positive, dated, enforceable and have the support of the administration as well as the staff. Review them periodically. It's perfectly appropriate to change these policies and procedures as the organization or medical treatments change.

After creating the manual, it's important to present it to the staff appropriately. Team members should be encouraged to participate in manual development and revision. Present it to the staff with this in mind: "These are the goals and objectives of our organization. The policies and procedures in this manual are to help *all of us* to understand our part in accomplishing these goals." Everyone should be familiar with the manual and instructed on new policies and procedures.

The ambulance service's manual is an indispensable link in the chain of providing quality patient care. It outlines the functions of the service as a whole and the team members individually and can be referred to and used to measure performance. It provides a means of communicating with employees and is a fair method for dealing with problems that may arise.

C A S E   S T U D Y   # 7

Service Improvement

Medic Ambulance Service crews are spending too much time on the scene of major-trauma cases. This was discovered by the medical director while reviewing trip sheets. He noted crews were spending on average 20 minutes at the scene of major-trauma patients. He knew this time had to be reduced and went to the manager to discuss the problem.

The medical director explained to the manager that the national standard for prehospital trauma management had changed and that short on-scene time was being stressed. Both the manager and the medical director believed that the long scene times were a system problem and not a fault of people within the organization. They called a meeting of the field supervisors to discuss the problem.

Medical director: "I called this meeting to discuss a problem I discovered while doing the monthly trip audits. We're spending too much time at the scene of major trauma patients—an average of 20 minutes. While I understand that although the concept of short on-scene time is somewhat new, the fact remains we need to reduce this time."

Ambulance manager: "The medical director and I felt that since you see the crews running these calls, you could help identify the problem areas as well as provide potential solutions."

Field supervisor 1: "I've felt that our on-scene times were too long for a while now, and I think the biggest problem is the lack of standing orders. For example, if the patient needs an endotracheal tube, I have to call into the hospital first. It takes me no less that two minutes to contact the hospital and another two minutes to get the order for the tube."

Field supervisor 2: "I've seen the same thing happen, but there's another problem as well. If we want to transport a patient to a hospital other than the hospital the patient requests, we need to clear it through dispatch first. While I understand the reason for this in other situations, it really slows us down when the patient needs to go to the trauma center."

Medical director: "Let me address the first problem that was brought up. It's important that paramedics work closely with base-station physicians. Having you call in for orders increases our ability to handle the tough medical calls. It's important that medical control is involved in medical decision-making in the field."

Field supervisor 1: "I agree. I think one of the strengths of this system is our working relationship with the medical director, but in this case, as opposed to a medical case, the radio call is not helping the patient. What if we set some standing orders for major trauma patients and then made sure that each and every one of these calls were reviewed closely by the medical director? I think this would help keep the good medical control this system is known for and allow us to treat the patient in a shorter amount of time."

Medical director: "What if we just did everything in the ambulance while transporting the patient to the hospital?"

Field supervisor 3: "We've been trying to do more of that, but that won't reduce the time lag we have from the time we see the patient until the time we can start IVs or intubate the patient. I think standing orders is a good idea. We've all gotten into the mind set of contacting the hospital at the scene, getting the orders, then loading the patient. I think between the standing orders and doing more in the ambulance we can reduce the on-scene time a lot."

Medical director: "I'll draw up a draft of a standing order for major-trauma patients. I'd like this group to review it before I take it to the physicians' advisory board for approval. I'll also talk to Dr. Smith who is head of the trauma-surgery department and see if she has any suggestions."

Ambulance manager: "Good, now let's address the problem of hospital destination. We instituted the call in policy to reduce the number of complaints we were getting from the patient's physician when we would change hospital destination. I felt that if we reduced the number of times it occurred and set a system to make sure the private physician was notified when it did happen, it would solve that problem. In fact it's been working well."

Field supervisor 2: "It may have helped there, but it's slowing us down on trauma calls. Often the trauma center is not the patient's regular hospital and his family doesn't understand that the patient needs to go there."

Ambulance manager: "Well, I'm willing to change the policy so it'll allow for a different approach when it's a trauma case. I'll rewrite the policy and we can review it when we review the new protocol. I'd like to thank you all for your help in this matter and look forward to seeing you at the next meeting."

■ ■ ■

Developing Accountability

Overview

Now that you've created a solid foundation and framework for the service, it's necessary to describe specific steps to make it work. As has been previously emphasized, an organization's most important organizational resource is its personnel. People are neither machines nor commodities. Much of this manual has been directed toward encouraging managers to use the personal touch with their staff. Yet, many managers adopt the mushroom philosophy of management: "Keep 'em in the dark and feed 'em manure." Most individuals are unhappy in this atmosphere. It certainly doesn't encourage performance.

A manager's expectations go a long way in determining team performance. Behavioral psychologists have often demonstrated this. Here's an example. Twenty adult students were enrolled in a class. The subject of the class isn't important, but it did involve learning difficult information and techniques. Unknown to the instructor, a few of the class members were *randomly* selected. These few students had no

(continued on next page)

(continued)

special intelligence or experience, but the instructor was *told* they showed a much higher aptitude for the course skills and content. The only thing different about them was the instructor's *perception and expectation* of the "better" students. What do you think the results were at the end of the course? These few elite students showed a higher level of proficiency and understanding of the course content. The only variable in the situation was the instructor's expectations. This same experiment has been repeated in a number of situations from elementary education to high-level management training. The lesson to be learned is obvious. The more you expect from individuals, the higher their performance.

INDIVIDUAL ACCOUNTABILITY

Ambulance services don't employ children to provide high-quality medical care. They employ adults. Therefore, managers should expect adult behavior and responsibility from their staff. Hold each member accountable, not only for their work, but for their behavior as well. Again, be positive, not negative. Your expectations will be rewarded. On the other hand, it you expect little from your team, that's what you'll get. You can't rely on "I told you they couldn't do it." The manager may fail by not having high expectations.

On the other hand, a manager can't expect everything to come from the staff automatically. Each team player must have the *authority* to take the action necessary to meet expectations. If the team member doesn't have this latitude to make decisions to improve personal performance, how can he exceed the expectations? At the same time, someone with authority to make personal decisions must be held *accountable* for those actions. This is a description of maturity. All of us are responsible for the decisions we make and the behavior that results.

Accountability holds an important place in EMS. Since many field personnel act without direct supervision, they must be held accountable for their actions. Other areas of operation, such as equipment and vehicle maintenance, also lend themselves to individual accountability.

Let's look at an example. Every time you turn around, more and more stethoscopes are missing or broken. At $36.50 apiece, this is no small matter. You can't keep replacing stethoscopes and still buy those new anti-shock trousers that are desperately needed. A stethoscope is used on every call and the trousers are needed only occasionally. Is there anything you can do to prevent this from happening again? What options are available?

Develop individual accountability. Buy enough stethoscopes for everyone. Yes, this is more expensive at first. But wait. Tell each paramedic that, under normal wear and tear, his stethoscope is expected to last two years. Each person is responsible for taking care of his own stethoscope. If it has to be replaced before the two years are up, the employee will have to pay for all or part of the cost of a new one. Of course, there may be special circumstances which can be dealt with on an individual basis but, as a rule, field personnel will be held accountable. Even though the initial expense may be higher, the overall cost of replacing stethoscopes will drop significantly. Each member will be more likely to take care of his own equipment, and repair costs will be reduced. This same procedure works well with other pieces of equipment as well.

The method of individual accountability can be considered a *negative* approach. But it works and is appropriate for many smaller pieces of equipment. If something accidental occurs, however, it shouldn't place the employee in financial jeopardy. That's not the policy's intent. The intent is to improve the care of the service's equipment.

Can this method of accountability be used for larger pieces of equipment such as ambulances? Yes and no. If you wrecked an ambulance, could you replace it from your savings account? It's doubtful! But it's still good to develop an accountability program. Let's look at a *positive* approach to create accountability for ambulances. There are two levels of responsibility to consider when requesting vehicle accountability. First, there must be individual responsibility for each vehicle. If all of the team members drive all of the ambulances, the personal sense of responsibility is diluted. A single individual or crew should be responsible for the same vehicle on each shift. Limit shifting of crews between vehicles. This will help establish a feeling of ownership. People take care of their own property better than they take care of other people's. The individual crews assigned to a specific rig should be held accountable for making sure the vehicle is mechanically sound, clean and restocked. They are responsible for reporting mechanical problems and making sure that the problems are corrected in an appropriate and timely manner. This ownership increases the crew's awareness and sense of responsibility. One beneficial side effect of accountability is that the drivers tend to be more careful and less prone to driving the wheels off the rigs. There's usually a marked improvement in vehicle appearance and maintenance as well.

POSITIVE REINFORCEMENT FOR THE TEAM

The other level of responsibility is group accountability, and it can be positively reinforced by management. Vehicle and equipment replacement and repair costs use a lot of the organization's financial resources. What if these expenses could be considerably reduced? Would the organization be willing to share the cost benefit? If so, you have a way to positively reinforce accountability. Many services reward exceptional actions for taking care of vehicles and equipment through financial incentives. Let's say that a service expects an ambulance to last five years. It costs $10,000 a year for those five years to pay for the ambulance. If a new ambulance is purchased after five years, the $10,000 per-year payments will continue. If the old ambulance can be used for another year, then the service can save that $10,000. If the service saves money because of the employees' exceptional efforts, how about sharing the wealth? Subtract any maintenance which would not be performed on a new vehicle. Maybe that will leave an $8,000 savings. Share some of it with the employees to reward their performance! This reward can be direct. The company could give 25 percent of the savings to the employees as a cash bonus. If your service is a government agency or doesn't allow such incentives, there are other ways to reward excellence. Maybe there's a piece of equipment team members would like to have. How about new carpeting in the day room, or a new TV set or a VCR? Don't stifle your creative juices. New uniforms, sending personnel to conferences, new radios, a picnic—any of these will provide new incentives and a feeling of satisfaction for a job well-done.

INVENTORY AND EQUIPMENT ACCOUNTABILITY

Inventory control prevents loss and ensures an adequate supply of material. What do you, as manager, want from an inventory system? You want to make sure patients are charged for the supplies they use. You want to know how much inventory is on hand and how much it's worth. And, finally, you want to make sure the service has enough supplies and equipment available to properly run the service.

Ambulance services should normally have two separate inventory listings. One list contains all of the service's re-useable equipment—medical, office, furniture, etc. The other list contains the expendable supplies for patient care or office use. We'll look at each type of inventory and discuss procedures for keeping track of the items.

■ Equipment inventory

Every re-usable item purchased by the service should be logged into the equipment-inventory ledger. Office calculators, staplers, traction splints, C-collars, tools, drug boxes, desks and radio batteries are but a few of the examples which fall into this category. The ledger log is a means of keeping track of all of these purchases. It can be divided into separate sections—one for medical equipment, one for maintenance equipment and one for office equipment. This helps to find an individual item later.

The log's format is simple. Each item is given a number and the item's description and serial number listed beside it. The date received and purchase price follow. Other helpful information may be listed, such as information on warranties, expected replacement dates and vendors. Figure 4.1 gives an example of what this log might look like.

Figure 4.1   Equipment Inventory

Criss Cross Ambulance Service Durable Equipment Inventory									
#	Description	Serial#	DateRec'd	Purch.Price	Warr.Exp.	Vendor	Log?	Loc.	Rep.Date
M-101	Traction splint	EE-135789	8/20/85	$109.00	8/26/86	EMT Supply	X	006	8/20/88
M-102	Extrication Collar Lg.	55432	8/25/87	$23.50	N/A	Mount. Sup.		003	8/25/88
M-103									

As you can see by the example, there's a lot of information that can be useful to you at a later date. The items are numbered sequentially as you receive them. In this example, the M at the beginning of the number differentiates medical equipment from office or shop equipment.

It's wise to make some kind of notation about warranties. For example, if a monitor battery fails, it's easy to look back in the inventory log to see if it's still under warranty and when that warranty expires. By including the vendor in the log, it'll be easier to find the original invoice or PO for warranty repair or replacement. It'll also help when items need replacing.

The last three columns are optional, but it makes it easier to have this information readily accessible. Many pieces of equipment will require preventative maintenance or corrective repair. The column marked "log?" asks the question whether or not a maintenance log has been prepared for that particular item. A maintenance log is a form used to document any routine maintenance, record who did it and when, record any repairs to the item and the cost incurred. By creating and using these maintenance logs, the manager can determine exactly how much each piece of equipment will cost to use over its lifetime. It will also help determine when it's necessary to replace the item. Another advantage of a maintenance log is that it documents care and checking. Many pieces of medical equipment must function within specific requirements. If a service doesn't periodically check these requirements and failure then occurs, there could be liability exposure for the organization.

If an item is assigned to a particular person, vehicle, office, station or other location, this can be noted in the location column. This makes it easier to find a particular piece of equipment when necessary. The final column includes the date that the piece of equipment is scheduled for replacement. It will help determine if the item should be repaired or replaced if it malfunctions at a later date.

A final column, which is not demonstrated in the figure, would provide for the disposition of equipment when it's no longer in the service's possession. This column would provide room for a statement of what happened to the equipment and when it should no longer be included in the service's inventory. For example, it might state "sold for $50—7/23/84" or "lost 5/13/83" or "discarded 3/3/83." This is important for accounting and inventory-value determination.

When a piece of equipment is entered in the inventory log, it's necessary to affix an inventory number to the item. This allows you to keep track of a specific item for as long as it's used by the service. This should be permanently painted, engraved, embossed or otherwise affixed—with no exceptions. Mark the name of the service or logo on the item. This will make it possible for someone to return the item if it's lost or left at a hospital.

Conduct once-a-year inventories to determine whether or not there are any missing pieces which might have gone undetected. It's time consuming but necessary. The location column on the inventory log will help. Any missing items should be marked as missing in the disposition column along with the date. At this time, an effort should be made by the entire team to locate these AWOL items.

■ Expendable supply inventory

It's far more difficult to keep track of expendable or disposable supplies. Generally, these supplies are divided into medical supplies, janitorial supplies and office supplies. The medical supplies consist of bandages, oxygen masks, disposable humidifiers, endotracheal tubes, tape, syringes and all other disposable patient-care items. This is the largest category of disposable inventory for ambulance services. The number of items may range from 40 to 50 for a small BLS service to a few hundred for a sophisticated ALS service. Unless an inventory system is installed, it'll be impossible to keep track of these items. In addition to assuring that supplies are always available for patients, the inventory system should reduce the amount of supplies that are wasted, lost or not charged to the patient.

The inventory system keeps track of supplies and shows the value of the supplies in the inventory. Can a system be developed, or is there a system available to do all of these things? Yes, but it takes time and a team effort for the system to work.

The first thing to do is to recruit one person who will be responsible for all disposable inventory. Give him the authority to prepare orders and establish procedures for taking supplies from the supply room. This is an important job which will take a lot of time. Therefore, extra compensation or a reduction of other responsibilities should accompany the duty.

Initially, take a complete inventory. It's usually necessary to assign a supply code number to each item in the inventory. This makes it possible to create order out of the existing chaos and to computerize your inventory when *and if* it's feasible. But in this manual we're going to discuss the old do-it-by-hand method. It works just as well and provides the same results as automated systems.

First, create a card or page for each item in the inventory book. This will be where the inventory specialist keeps track of each item. Many office-supply companies have pre-printed inventory cards which work well. The use of the information on this card will determine how well your system will work. The information which is included on the inventory card is detailed below.

Item number. The item number is the number you assign to each item in the supply inventory. The actual number chosen isn't important, but first it's a good idea to arrange the supply room in some logical order. The different types and sizes of tape should be in one place, bandaging supplies nearby, syringes and IV supplies in the same general area. Group oxygen masks, cannulas and other airway supplies together. This makes it easier to find each item and creates order in the supply room.

When assigning numbers to similar items of various sizes, number them accordingly. For example, oral airways come in various sizes. Therefore, assign the smallest number to the smallest airway, and the largest number to the largest airway. Size 0 airway might have number M-3000, size 1 might be assigned M-3010, size 2—M-3020 and so on. It's a good idea *not* to number items consecutively because then you can later inject new inventory items into the system and not lose numerical order. If a new airway were to be included in the system which was considered size 1½ and you had numbered size 1 as M-3003 and size 2 as M3002, where would you put size 1½? With the earlier numbering system, however, size 1½ would fit nicely into the M-3015 slot.

Item description. Once you've organized the stockroom and assigned inventory numbers to the supplies, fill in the description blank. Simply tell what the item is, and include the size if different sizes are in stock. That's the easy part. There's another important part of the description. Medical supplies are ordered in different quantities—by item, bottle, box or case. Other units are also possible. It's impossible to remember exactly how many units are in each quantity ordered. Do you know how many 5″ × 9″ dressings are in a case? How many boxes of 4″ × 4″s are in a case? Different size solutions have a different number of units in each case.

Therefore, in addition to describing the item, it's a good idea to include information about how the units were packaged. For example, let's say that 4″ × 4″ gauze dressings are ordered by the case. There might be 1000 individual dressings in a case. Sterile 4″ × 4″s usually come two to a package. There might be 50 packages to a box and 10 boxes to a case. All of this information is necessary for inventory and reordering, but it's too much information to write in that little description blank. There's a shorthand method you can use: 10 Bx [50 Pkg (2 Ea/Pkg)]/Cs. This simply says there are two each to a package, 50 packages to a box, and 10 boxes to a case. Fortunately, most items are easier to describe. Endotracheal tubes simply come in 10 Ea./Bx. IV solutions might be 12 bags/Cs. An item ordered by the unit is described as Ea.

Vendors. In the space provided, list two or three of the vendors from whom the items are ordered. Identify the primary vendor. This will help when the orders are prepared. The individual in charge of inventory can create a separate order form for the different vendors.

Unit cost. List the unit cost of the item for each vendor. The unit cost is the cost of *one* item or package. In the example about 4″ × 4″s, the unit would be a package. You can't use just one 4″ × 4″ and save the other one in the package, because once the package is opened, anything left is thrown away. For inventory, match the unit cost with how each item is counted. To determine unit cost it may be necessary to divide the cost of the ordered quantity (for example, a case) by the number of units in the overall quantity. For 4″ × 4″s, the unit cost would be the cost of a case divided by 500 packages.

Minimum balance. The minimum balance is the lowest quantity you want stocked. This is determined by how frequently the items are used, how long it takes to get an order and how often you order. If you order supplies once a month, you'll need a minimum supply of two or three months in stock. If a minimum is reached shortly after supplies are ordered, it'll be a month before they'll be ordered. Also remember that there'll be some time between the time you order and when you actually get the items. Therefore, a buffer is needed in case delivery is delayed, the items are back ordered or you use more than you anticipated. A two-month supply might be conservative but is generally sufficient.

Maximum balance. This is the quantity your inventory shouldn't exceed. A 10-year supply of bedpans isn't needed so why tie up all that money? Remember to allow for the amount you'll be ordering. A maximum of 1000 for 4″ × 4″s wouldn't be appropriate. If you order one case, you get 1000. That means in order to not exceed your maximum allowance you'll have to wait until you're out of stock. It won't work. Depending on use, 1250 to 1500 might be a better number.

That way when the inventory clerk finds there's a quarter of a case left, a new case can be ordered, and the maximum not exceeded. In this example, the minimum for 4″ × 4″s would be 250 (or one-quarter case).

Balance on hand. From the careful inventory you've completed, you know how many items are on hand. Fill this amount into the balance-on-hand location for the month. Easy enough! But don't waste your employees' time by demanding accounting for every item. We don't count every Band-Aid, but we do count every box and case. For example, there might be four half boxes of Band-Aids for inventory purposes. On the other hand, if the service charges for each individual Band-Aid, it'll be necessary to count each one. The general rule when counting inventory is to count each item if it's charged or dispensed on a per-unit basis.

Date. This is simply the date that the items were counted.

Number used. This is the number of items used or dispensed in the previous month. The number used is the difference between the balance on hand for the current month and the previous month's balance.

Date and number ordered. When the inventory clerk determines it's time to reorder, the date and quantity ordered is entered on each of the item cards for the supplies ordered. This will prevent double ordering, and lets everyone know that the item should be received shortly.

Date and number received. When the supplies are received and added to the inventory, the number and the date received should be added to the cards. The balance then can be updated during the next cycle to show the increased supply.

Number back ordered. If only part of the ordered items are received, or if the vendor notifies the service that the item has been back ordered, this is noted on the item card. This will let the person handling inventory know that the item has already been ordered and why it hasn't been received.

This inventory method allows the service to keep track of its supplies and prevents running out of needed items. But it doesn't really keep track of the supplies that leave the storeroom. There are different procedures for keeping track of such supplies. Often, no procedure is used. The crews simply go into the storeroom and get what they need to replace supplies on the ambulance. This leaves a hole in the system because nobody knows what's actually happening to the supplies. There are two ways to control this. One is informal—a sign-out sheet. All items taken from the storeroom are listed and signed for by the person who removes them. This works in some services, but it doesn't completely solve the problem. An informal system might be appropriate if the service can determine the specific number of items charged, and can then compare those numbers to the numbers listed as used on the monthly inventory report. If the discrepancy is small, the manager may decide to keep an informal system.

■ Treating each unit as a cost center

Keep a manifest and update it each time the vehicle changes crews. The manifest lists every item and its quantity on board the ambulance. As an item is used, it's listed on the manifest. At the end of the shift, the crew takes the manifest to the supply person and gets replacement supplies on a one-for-one basis. Figure 4.2 is a copy of a vehicle manifest.

These manifests are taken to the office daily and compared with the run reports and patient charges listed by the crew after their runs. This is an effective way to make sure that each item used is charged and that no supplies slip through the crack. If items are used but not charged, the crew lists them on the manifest along with the reason. The items might have been used in a training session, wasted, lost, damaged or used on a patient who was not transported or charged. This method is by far the best, but it takes more time and effort.

With this system, determining the value of the supplies on hand (your inventory) is not difficult. The *manifest* identifies the amount of supplies on each vehicle and the *monthly inventory* keeps track of the supplies in the storeroom. The easist way to determine the value of the inventory is to take the numbered items on hand (in the storeroom and in the vehicles) and multiply that quantity by the unit cost. After adding all of these together, you have the overall value of your inventory.

CORRECTIVE VS. PREVENTIVE MAINTENANCE

Once you establish individual accountability, create programs and procedures to help the team follow through. Maintenance programs have two purposes. To make sure that a vehicle or piece of equipment is available and functioning *properly* when needed, and to extend the life of the vehicle or equipment.

In an EMS system, the first purpose is by far the most important. Much of the technologically sophisticated equipment on ambulances leaves little room for error. They must perform flawlessly each time they're used. Therefore, it's necessary to have an exacting maintenance program. The same is true for vehicles. If your team doesn't get there, it can't do the job. Beware of trying to extend the useful life of a vehicle, or any piece of equipment, beyond reason. The money saved is false economy. For example, you try to squeeze an extra two years out of your defibrillator, it fails at the wrong time with the wrong patient and the cost of the lawsuit could have bought 1,000 new defibrillators. Likewise, damage done to your public image resulting from long response times because of ambulance mechanical failures costs more than the price of a new vehicle. If you give your team broken bats, don't expect them to get very many hits, let alone win the game.

When thinking of maintenance programs, think of the space program. There's no room for error. Your vehicles and equipment *must* perform when needed. Each piece of equipment must be maintained and cleaned. Even though each piece probably has its own peculiarities and specific requirements, these procedures need to be done on a regular basis and accountability must be established. Any good maintenance program will have the following elements:

Discovery. Uncover any problem or malfunction before, not during, an ambulance call or other critical situation.

Reporting. Report the problem to the person responsible for correcting the situation.

Corrective action. Correct the problem through replacement or repair.

Feedback. Tell the person who reported the problem that it's been corrected.

Monitoring. Monitor the results to determine if the program is working efficiently and to account for expenses.

Ideally, problems (broken equipment, vehicle malfunction, and so on) are discovered through routine procedures. The vehicle and equipment checklist is the most efficient way to review equipment status. Each oncoming crew carefully checks their equipment and vehicle against a standardized checklist, which makes the job easier and more efficient. There's less chance of overlooking details. An example of the checklist is included (see Figures 4.2 and 4.3).

Figure 4.2 Vehicle Manifest (front)

DAILY SHIFT REPORT

Date _____ Unit _____

CREW CHANGES —

_____ for _____

Out _____ Reason _____

Out _____ for _____

Out _____ Reason _____

Out _____

Out _____ Special Event _____

Out _____ Holiday Hours _____

CREW —

EMT : In _____ Out _____

EMT-P : In _____ Out _____

SECOND CREW —

EMT : In _____ Out _____

EMT-P : In _____ Out _____

THIRD CREW —

EMT : In _____ Out _____

EMT-P : In _____ Out _____

RUN NO.	TIME OUT	RUN NO.	TIME OUT	RUN NO.	TIME OUT	RUN NO.	TIME OUT	LATE RUN NO.

INCIDENT COMPLAINT

NO. _____ NATURE _____

FUEL TICKETS

Receipt No.	Gal.	Cost

EQUIPMENT FAILURE

EFR No.	Type of Equipment

ACCIDENT REPORT

REVIEWED BY _____

ADDITIONAL NARRATIVE: _____

EQUIPMENT —

Apcor

Walki-talkie

Life Pak 5

Laerdal suction

Drug box (adult)

Drug box (ped)

Trauma kit A

Trauma kit B

Burn pac

Active-aid board

Active-aid board

MAST pants (adult)

MAST pants (ped)

Sager splint

Sager splint

Pro-splint kit (ped)

Pro-splint kit (adult)

KED board

KED board

EQUIPMENT —

C-collar Thomas (adult) (4)

C-collar Thomas (adult) (4)

C-collar Thomas (ped) (4)

C-collar Thomas (ped) (4)

PMR bag (adult)

PMR bag (ped)

Portable 02 — PSI

Installed 02 — PSI

Extra portable 02 tanks (2)

Flo-meters (2)

Sandbags 5-lbs.

Sandbags 10-lbs.

Primary stretcher

Stair chair

Scoop stretcher

Folding stretchers

Fire extinguisher (2)

Flares (4)

Map book

Trash can

Trash bags

Observer helmet

DRIVER'S NAME	START MILES	END MILES	START #30's	END #30's	START #50's	END #50's	NUMBER OF CALLS

EMT SIGNATURE _____

PARAMEDIC SIGNATURE _____

OFF-GOING PARAMEDIC _____

Figure 4.3 Vehicle Manifest (back)

Supply	Unit	Ad Box	AWB	TB 1	TB 2	Total	Inventory Used	ADJ
Oral Airways: 40mm	1		1	1	1	4		
Oral Airways: 60mm	1		1	1	1	4		
Oral Airways: 80mm	1		1	1	1	4		
Oral Airways: 90mm	1		1	1	1	4		
Oral Airways: 100mm	1		1	1	1	4		
Nasal Airways: sz 6.0mm	1		1	1	1	4		
Nasal Airways: sz 7.0mm	1		1	1	1	4		
Nasal Airways: sz 8.0mm	1		1	1	1	4		
ET Tubes (ped) sz 3.0	1		1			2		
ET Tubes (ped) 3.5	1		1			2		
ET Tubes (ped) sz 4.0	1		1			2		
ET Tubes sz 5.0	1		1			2		
ET Tubes (ped) sz 6.0	1		1			2		
ET Tubes sz 6.0	1		1			2		
ET Tubes sz 7.0	1		1			2		
ET Tubes sz 8.0	1		1			2		
ET Tubes sz 9.0	1		1			2		
ET Styletts 1 ea adult & ped	1ea	1ea				2		
EOA Kits	1		1	1	1	4		
EOA Tubes	2					2		
Disp Bulb Syringe	1		1			2		
Delee Suction	3		1			4		
Epinephrine 1:1,000	2	2				4		
Epinephrine 1:10,000	4	5				9		
Sodium Bicarb 50cc	7	5				12		
Atropine 1mg	4	2				6		
Lidocaine 100mg	2	1				3		
Lidocaine 2 Gr	2					2		
Calcium Chloride 1 Gr	3	3				6		
Dextrose 50%	2	2				4		
Lasix 40mg	2	4				6		
Bretylium 500mg	4	4				8		
Isuprel 1mg	2	2				4		
Intropin 400mg	1	1				2		
Narcan 0.4mg	2	4				6		
Nitro Tablets	3btl	1btl				4		
Ipecac 30cc	3	2				5		
Glucose Paste	2	2				4		
Ammonia Inhalants	1bx	1bx				2bxs		

Supply	Unit	Ad Box	AWB	TB 1	TB 2	Total	Inventory Used	ADJ
LR 250ml	4	1				5		
LR 500ml	4	1				5		
LR 1,000ml	4		3	3		10		
D5W 250ml	4					10		
Med Labels	5	5				10		
Tubes Syringe	1	1				2		
Butterflys 23ga	1	1				2		
Butterflys 25ga	1	1				2		
Needle 21ga	6	6				12		
Regular Drip	7	1	3	3		14		
Mini Drip	7	2				9		
Syringes 1cc	2	1				3		
Syringes 3cc	2	1				3		
Syringes 6cc	4	1	1			6		
Syringes 12cc	4	1	1			6		
Syringes 35cc	2	1				3		
IV Catheter 24ga	1					1		
IV Catheter 22ga	6	2				8		
IV Catheter 20ga	6	4				10		
IV Catheter 18ga	6	4	3	3		16		
IV Catheter 16ga	6	4	3	3		16		
IV Catheter 14ga	6	4	3	3		16		
Buretrol	1	1				2		
Tourniquets	2	5	2	2		8		
Alcohol Wipes	100	12	10	10		132		
Padded Arm Board 3x18	2	1				3		
Padded Arm Board 2x9	2	1				3		
Bioclusive	6	4	4	4		18		
Finger Lances	12					12		
Dextrostiks	6					6		
Vacu Needles 21ga	6	6				12		
Red Top Tubes (adult)	1	1				2		
Vacu Holders (adult)	4	4				8		
Vacu Holders (ped)	1	1				2		
Red Top Tubes (ped)	4	4				8		
Cloth Tape 1"	2	1	1	1		6		
Dermiclear 1"	2	1	2	2		8		
4x4 Sterile	25	2	4	4		35		
5x9 Bandage	15	2	4	4		33		

Supply	Unit	Ad Box	AWB	TB 1	TB 2	Total	Inventory Used	ADJ
Multi-Trauma Dressing	5			2	2	9		
Thermometer	H 1	1				2		
Lubricating Jelly	12		10	4	4	30		
Electrode (adult)	bx	1pg				12pg		
Electrode (ped)	bx	3pg				12pg		
Tube of Defib Jelly	1					2		
Iodine Preps	bx	6				bx		
Triangular Bandage	3			1	1	5		
Kerlix	10	1		2	2	15		
Vaseline Gauze	bx					14		
Band-aids	bx	10				60		
Disp OB Kits	2					2		
Silver Swaddlers	2	1				3		
O2 Tubing	3					3		
O2 Mask (adult)	8		1			9		
Nasal Cannula (adult)	8					3		
O2 Mask w/NRB bag (adult)	3					4		
O2 Mask (ped)	3		1			4		
Nasal Cannula (ped)	4					5		
O2 Mask w/NRB bag (ped)	2		1			3		
Humidifier	2					2		
Premee Feeding Tube 5Fr	1					2		
Suction Catheter 8Fr	2	1				3		
Suction Catheter 14Fr	2	1				3		
Suction Catheter 14Fr	3					3		
Replacement Suction Bag	3					3		
Tonsil Tip	3	1				4		
Suction Tubing	3					4		
EKG Paper	3rl					pak		
4x4 Non-sterile	pak					pak		
Ice Paks	4					4		
H2O Sterile	3					3		
NS Sterile	3					3		
Sharps Receptacle	1					1		
Ladder Splints	3					3		
Zip-lock Bags	6					6		
Cast Bucket	4					4		
Box of Tissue	2					2		
Burn Sheet	2					2		

Supply	Unit	Ad Box	AWB	TB 1	TB 2	Total	Inventory Used	ADJ
Chucks	10					10		
Disp Mask	bx					bx		
Non-sterile Gloves	bx					bx		
Pillow	2					2		
Blankets	2					2		
Sheets	10					10		
Pillow Cases	6					6		
Towels	1pg					1pg		

Equipment	Unit	Ad Box	AWB	TB 1	TB 2	Total	ADJ
Laryngoscope Handle	1		1			2	
Wis-hipple sz 1	1			1	1	1	
Miller sz 4	1					2	
Miller sz 2	1					2	
McIntosh sz 4	1					2	
1 Large Bulb	1					2	
1 Small Bulb	1					2	
C-cell Batteries	2					4	
McGill (adult)	1					2	
McGill (ped)							
Stethoscope (adult)	1			1	1	3	
Stethoscope (ped)	1					1	
S/R Stethoscope (adult)	1					1	
Ped Kit for S/R Steth	1					4	
BP Cuff (adult)	1		1	1	1	4	
BP Cuff (child set)	1					1	
BP Thigh Cuff	1					1	
PMR Bag (ped) w/mask			1			1	
PMR Bag (adult) w/mask			1			1	

Create a standardized format for reporting a situation to the person responsible for correcting it. The form in Figure 4.4 will help. The particular equipment item or vehicle is identified and the problem clearly explained. The person responsible for corrective action can then prepare a work order and make sure that the work is undertaken. This work order should also be prepared to help obtain bids and record costs. Once the repairs are done and inspected by the person responsible for the correction, send a memo to the team member who reported the problem. This feedback reassures that person *and* the entire team that problems reported are heard and corrected. If records are well-kept and complete, the staff will be better able to keep track of the maintenance history of each vehicle and equipment item. The cost and number of repairs for each item will help determine when each item should be replaced or if it's not cost-effective.

ADVANTAGES OF PREVENTIVE MAINTENANCE

The procedure above describes a *corrective* maintenance program. Better yet is a *preventive* maintenance program. The object is to prevent failure and malfunction, not just to correct it once it's occurred. In a preventive maintenance program, each item and vehicle undergoes periodic inspection and maintenance designed to prevent failures. The manufacturers of most equipment used by EMS services supply information on routine care. This information, as well as other common-sense procedures, should be written down in the services's inventory for each item. Individual team members should be responsible for examining these pieces of equipment periodically and performing the routine maintenance. Again, accountability is important. Document and date the servicing of each piece of equipment. The documentation can then be reviewed to ensure compliance. Even though vehicles are more complicated and routine care is more involved, they should be serviced in the same manner. Periodic care will improve their reliability and extend their useful life. The appendix includes a list of some of the procedures for vehicle and equipment preventive maintenance. A good preventive maintenance program will *save* money. It will also improve morale. Nothing is more frustrating to a paramedic than an equipment failure

Figure 4.4 Equipment Failure/Problem Report

EQUIPMENT FAILURE/PROBLEM REPORT No. 1

UNIT NO.	DATE PROBLEM REPORTED		VEHICLE ID #
	MONTH	DAY	YEAR

SENIOR CREW MEMBER:	DRIVER DURING SHIFT THIS REPORT WAS MADE:

VEHICLE/EQUIPMENT FAILURE DISCOVERED
(Check only one box in this section)

| NOT DURING ASSIGNED RUN | ☐ DURING SHIFT CHECKOUT |
| | ☐ OTHER (Describe) |

| DURING ASSIGNED RUN | ☐ EN ROUTE | RUN NO. |
| | ☐ AT SCENE | |

TIME CREW AFFECTED

TIME FAILURE REPORTED:

TIME CREW (Check one)	☐ Taken out of service
	☐ Unavailable as 1st responder
TIME CREW BACK IN SERVICE- ALL PRIORITIES (Check one)	☐ Same equipment vehicle
	☐ Different equipment vehicle
TOTAL TIME: (Check one)	☐ Crew out of service
	☐ Crew unavailable as 1st responder

THIS EQUIPMENT PROBLEM ☐ DID / ☐ DID NOT INTERRUPT AN AMBULANCE RUN IN PROGRESS

TYPE OF FAILURE   Check box and describe failure in comments section

MILEAGE:

☐ Accidents
☐ Body Cab Misc.
☐ Glass Mirrors
☐ Wipers Blades
☐ AM FM radio
☐ Heater Front Rear
☐ Defroster
☐ Air Cond. Front Rear
☐ Seats and Seat Belts
☐ Door and Hinges

☐ Chassis Misc.
☐ Brakes
☐ Service Parking
☐ Springs
☐ Shocks
☐ Steering
☐ Alignment
☐ Wheels
☐ Tires

☐ Cooling Misc.
☐ Water Pump
☐ Radiator
☐ Hoses Radiator Heater
☐ Belts

☐ Electrical Misc.
☐ Alternator
☐ Regulator
☐ Starter
☐ Battery L R
☐ Turn Signals L R
☐ Brake Lights
☐ Hazard Lights

☐ Back Up Lights
☐ Headlights Hi Lo
☐ Headlight Flasher
☐ Fog Lights
☐ Spot Lights L R
☐ Light Bar
☐ Strobes Pri Sec
☐ Cowl Beacons
☐ Scene Lights L R Rear
☐ Auto Throttle
☐ Siren W. y. h-l. pa. elec. air manual. radio speaker
☐ Horn
☐ Air Horn
☐ Int. Lights Hi-Lo Dome Att. Panel
☐ Suction Rear Vent
☐ Shore Line
☐ 110 Vac Recp. Interior PDQ Panel
☐ 110 Heater Battery Cond.
☐ GFCI On Off Trip

☐ Drive Train Misc.
☐ Transmission
☐ Drive Shaft
☐ Differential
☐ Rear Axles
☐ Engine Misc.
☐ PM
☐ Idle Smooth Rough
☐ Exhaust Misc Leak
☐ Mufflers
☐ Glow Plugs
☐ Injection
☐ Injection Pump

VEHICLE RADIO
FRONT CONTROL HEADS
☐ Switches
☐ Lights
☐ Transmit Receive
 ☐ Channel _____ t r
 ☐ Channel _____ t r
☐ Other
REAR CONTROL HEAD
☐ Switches
☐ Lights
☐ Transmit Receive
☐ ECG Calibration
☐ Intercom Operation
☐ Other
PORTABLE RADIO MX
ID #
MEDICAL TELEMETRY RADIO
☐ Steering
☐ Transmit Receive
☐ Other
HANDIE TALKIE HT
ID #
☐ Transmit Receive
☐ Other
PAGER
ID #
☐ Tone
☐ Voice
☐ Other
ALERT MONITOR
ID #
☐ Tone
☐ Voice
☐ Other

ID #
BRAND

☐ Airway Bag
☐ Ambu Bag (Adult)
☐ Ambu Bag (Pediatric)
☐ Laryngoscope Handle
☐ Laryngoscope Blade
☐ Backboard (Long)
☐ Backboard (Short)
☐ Burn Pack
☐ Cardioscope - Battery Charger
☐ Cardioscope - Case
☐ Cardioscope - Defibrillator
☐ Cardioscope - Lead Cables
☐ Cardioscope - Screen
☐ Cardioscope - Strip Recorder
☐ Drug Box
☐ Fire Extinguisher
☐ Oxygen Flow Meter
☐ Portable Oxygen - Rack
☐ Portable Oxygen - Tank
☐ Pneumatic Shock Trouser
☐ Sager Traction Splint
☐ Scoop Stretcher
☐ Sphygmomanometer (B.P. Cuff)
☐ Splint
☐ Stair Chair
☐ Stethoscope
☐ Stretcher (Primary)
☐ Stretcher (Secondary)
☐ Suction (In Dwelling)
☐ Suction (Portable)
☐ Trauma Bag
☐ Other

COMMENTS:

FOR CITY USE ONLY:	SENIOR CREW MEMBER SIGNATURE: **X**
Date white copy received:	

Mechanic Report (Vehicle) - Supervisor Report (Equipment)

DESCRIPTION OF REPAIRS REPLACEMENT SOLVING PROBLEM:

LIST CODES OF ACTUAL REPAIRS MADE:

WARRANTY IN-SHOP REPAIR OUT-OF-SHOP REPAIR	DATE REPAIRS COMPLETED OR EQUIPMENT RETURNED TO IN-SERVICE
Date pink copy received:	MECHANIC OR SUPERVISOR SIGNATURE: **X**

at a critical time. Services that show they care about equipment foster team pride and competence in patient care leading to a positive image in the community they serve.

RISK MANAGEMENT AND INSURANCE ISSUES

Each organization should annually review its insurance coverage for exposure to risks. Radical changes have taken place in the insurance industry in the past several years, with the need for and the cost of coverage increasing. Following are common types of coverage that services should have.

General:
   Vehicle liability
   General liability
   Comprehensive and physical damage for vehicles
   Property (general, fire, theft and commercial liability)
   Umbrella coverage
   Employee health

Professional:
   Directors' and officers' coverage
   Medical malpractice
   Performance bonding

The best buy for EMS organizations may be through group purchasing agreements, such as the one the American Ambulance Association sponsors for its members. These types of programs tend to be more competitive than shopping for coverage from a local agent or broker. This is because of the national buying power of the group and the specialized nature of the pool of participants. Because these types of insurance providers specialize in EMS and have experience in the industry, they are normally much easier to work with on claims and other related problems.

Reducing the risk of accidents, injury or other claims is an important part of the manager's job. With the increasing costs of insurance and the increasing number of lawsuits against health-care providers, the best way to protect the service is to prevent claims. Awareness and active research into risk management is a means by which ambulance insurance costs can be controlled or reduced.

SYSTEM ACCOUNTABILITY THROUGH IMPROVED PERSONNEL SCHEDULING

Scheduling personnel provides an interesting challenge for the manager. How you handle this task has a profound effect on the total system. Personnel scheduling directly affects response times, patient care and the financial success of the entire system.

For example, if too few crews are available to meet the demands of the system, response times will be unacceptably long. Crews that are expected to perform at high levels for long periods of time will be unable to deliver optimum patient care. Having too many people scheduled, or having too much overtime jeopardizes the service's financial well-being. This demonstrates why schedules must be carefully planned and developed and must not be a fill-in-the-hole process.

EMS scheduling can't be viewed in the traditional staffing manner. Creative and innovative ideas must be included to increase efficiency and effectiveness. The people who have chosen EMS as a career have not come to expect the traditional 40-hour work week, and for many services this is not a workable option. A combination of 24-hour, 12-hour, 10-hour, eight-hour and part-time peak-load shifts may be used within the same service to provide adequate coverage.

Every manager would like to have surplus crews available. Financial reality, however, makes that unrealistic in today's economy. To create an efficient staffing pattern, it's necessary to first identify the minimum amount of staffing required and then determine the maximum you can afford. Figure 2.9, Unit-Hour Analysis, helps to illustrate this (see page 97).

It's necessary for you as manager to learn and understand what goes into scheduling and the effect each staffing option has on the operations and finances of the organization. That's what you're paid for.

This staffing pattern would meet the minimum needs of the organization. With a total budget allowance of $225,000 for salaries, most managers would be tempted to staff another vehicle for 24 hours a day, for a total salary expense of $219,000. That leaves $6,000 in the salary budget. We can live with that—but can we? It's not so simple. There are other things to be considered. First, your service would be unique if all calls were evenly spaced over a 24-hour period to match your unit availability. It may be that more than two ambulances are needed during peak periods and fewer than two units during quiet early morning hours. That's not the only thing to consider. The Criss Cross EMTs are going to receive a salary of only $10,400 per year ($5.00 x 2080 hours per year). The paramedics will do a little better at $15,600. Is that going to be enough to attract and keep the best employees for Criss Cross? Another thing to think about is that some of the benefit expenses are disproportionate to the total salary, and instead determined by the number of employees. For example, health insurance, training costs, uniform allowances, sick leave, some retirement plans and vacations are determined by the number of employees and are not necessarily a percentage of the total salaries.

Innovative and alternative staffing structures are important in this industry. The call load, number of employees and employee-salary levels must all be considered in making staffing decisions. To outline alternatives, let's again review staffing of one vehicle for 24 hours a day for one year. But, instead of eight-hour shifts for the technicians, we'll look at a staffing pattern which has the crew members working 24 hours and off 48 hours.

One new definition needs to be introduced. The straight-time equivalent (STE) is the number of hours worked converted to straight-time pay. This provides a yardstick for measuring salary costs by a single unit. In the 24/48 shift pattern, each person works an average of 56 hours per week. Forty of those hours will be straight time and 16 will be overtime. (Yes, there are some ways to get around the overtime-pay requirements for 24-hour employees, but subtracting sleep time is hard to document and doesn't sit well with the staff. A better way to handle that is to keep the hourly rate artificially low, so the total take-home pay remains approximately the same. More about that later.) The straight-time equivalent for these employees will be 64 hours per week (40 hours + 1.5 x 16 hours). The annual wages for these 24/48 employees will be $16,640 for EMTs and $24,960 for paramedics.

Now to determine the total Criss Cross salary costs for the year. That's easy. Take the annual salary of each employee level and multiply it by the number of employees. Hold it! Eight and one half employees are no longer needed. With the 24/48 shift only six employees, three EMTs and three paramedics, are required.

$$\begin{aligned} \$16,640 \times 3 &= \quad \$49,920 \\ + \ \$24,960 \times 3 &= \quad \underline{\$74,880} \\ & \quad \ \ \$124,800 \end{aligned}$$

The difference between paying 8.5 employees, who work 40 hours a week, and six 24/48 employees is $15,300 per year. Maybe $15,000 doesn't look like much when all is considered. It depends on how much employee benefits are reduced because of the fewer number of employees. Also the cost of training new employees will more than likely be less. The more attractive salaries will go a long way in keeping the staff on board. The shifts longer than eight hours have many personal advantages to the employees and can do a lot for employee motivation and morale.

Let's continue to explore alternatives. The Criss Cross board of directors thought that $25,000 was too much to pay paramedics. They also thought it wasn't necessary to pay $16,000 + to attract qualified EMTs. But they did like the other advantages of the 24/48 hour shift. What could they do? What if the hourly wages were not set in stone? This might create a whole new set of opportunities for creative scheduling. They decided to see what would happen if they paid the EMTs $4.00 per hour and the paramedics $6.00. This is what they discovered:

$4.00 per hour × 64 STEs per week × 52 weeks = $13,312 for EMTs
$6.00 per hour × 64 STEs per week × 52 weeks = $19,968 for paramedics

$$\begin{array}{rl} \$13,312 \times 3 = & \$39,936 \\ + \ \$19,968 \times 3 = & \$59,904 \\ \hline & \$99,840 \end{array}$$

The Criss Cross board was happy. They had fewer employees, each receiving more money per year and the total salary cost to the service was nearly $25,000 less. They also would experience less cost for the benefits given to fewer employees. This is just one example of how creative staffing can solve difficult problems. But it barely touches the possibilities. What can Criss Cross do about the extra staffing needs? A second ambulance could be staffed with 24/48 crews and still leave $25,000 + in the budget to meet peak demands. That would be taking the easy way out. Other types of shifts could be reviewed to make sure that the staffing is applied to the times for which additional crews are needed. The same type of procedure demonstrated in the example above can be used to determine the *best* schedule for the other shifts. Combinations of 12-hour shifts and eight-hour shifts could be considered. Figure 4.5 provides you with examples of some of the unlimited variations of work schedules. Don't

Figure 4.5 Sample Work Schedule

AVG HRS/WK	HRS/ SHIFT	CYCLE LENGTH	R.T. HRS/CYCLE	O.T. HRS/CYCLE	AVG STE's PER WK	1	2	3	4	5	6	7	8	9	10	11	12	13	14	15	16	17	18	19	20	21
																										SCHEDULE GUIDE (DAYS)
84.00	24	4WKS	160	176	106.00	W	O	O	O					W	O	W	O									
84.00	24	2WKS	80	88	106.00	W	O																			
60.00	24	12WKS	448	224	65.33	O	O	O	W	O	O	O	O	O	O	W	O	W								
56.00	24	3WKS	120	48	64.00	W	O	O																		

(Other variations are available with the above pattern by scheduling "kelly" days or additional days off every 7 to 14 working days. This will give variations of 48 to 52 average hours per week.)

AVG HRS/WK	HRS/ SHIFT	CYCLE LENGTH	R.T. HRS/CYCLE	O.T. HRS/CYCLE	AVG STE's PER WK	1	2	3	4	5	6	7	8	9	10	11	12	13	14	15	16	17	18	19	20	21
56.00	24	9WKS	360	144	64.00	W	O	W	O	W	O	W	O	O												
50.40	24	10WKS	400	104	55.60	O	W	O	W	O	W	O	W	O	O											
46.67	24	18WKS	536	304	55.10	W	O	O	W	O	W	O	W	O	O	O	O	O	O	O	O	O				
42.00	24	4WKS	144	24	45.00	W	O	O	O																	
56.00	10/14	12WKS	462	210	64.75	10	10	10	10	14	14	14	14	O	O	O	O									
56.00	10/14	9WKS	360	144	64.00	10	10	10	14	14	14	O	O	O												
42.00	10/14	12WKS	450	54	44.25	10	10	10	O	O	O	14	14	14												
42.00	10/14	8WKS	304	32	44.00	10	10	10	14	14	O	O	O													

or

AVG HRS/WK	HRS/ SHIFT	CYCLE LENGTH	R.T. HRS/CYCLE	O.T. HRS/CYCLE	AVG STE's PER WK	1	2	3	4	5	6	7	8	9	10	11	12	13	14	15	16	17	18	19	20	21
42.00	12/12	8WKS	304	32	44.00	W	W	W	W	W	O	O	O	D	D	D	D	D	D	D	O	M	M	M		
41.00	8/8/8	4WKS	144	24	45.00	A	A	A	M	A	A	A	A	O					D	O	M	M	M	M	M	M
																			A=Afternoon D=Day M=Midnight							
40.00	8	1WKS	40	40	0.00	W	W	W	W	W	O	O	O													

Legend:

Cycle represents the period of time that a specific schedule requires before it repeats on the same day of the week.

STE are Straight Time Equivalents -- all overtime is figured at time-and-one-half.

All overtime is calculated on anything over 40hrs in one week.

The shift patterns listed under the schedule guide are repeated to produce the full schedule.

There are many variations possible for the presented schedules. This is produced only as a guide. The average STE determines the respective cost for each schedule.

be restricted. Think creatively! Your staff and your patients will thank you.

MISCELLANEOUS SCHEDULING

Wage and Hour. In 1985 the U.S. Supreme Court struck down an earlier decision which had excluded government agencies from adhering to many of the federal wage and hour regulations. This simply means that all organizations, public and private, must adhere to the wage and hour regulations regarding work weeks, overtime pay, salaried employees, and so on. Many ambulance districts, city ambulance services and county-run EMS organizations no longer are exempt from these regulations. But, it's expected these regulations will change several times in the next few years. It would be wise to make sure your organization complies with the law.

One point worth noting is that there are provisions in the regulations concerning 24-hour shifts. These provisions allow the employer not to pay his employee for a full 24 hours if the employer guarantees the employee a specified number of uninterrupted rest hours. Used by many services to control personnel costs, it should be avoided. Most employees dislike being at work and not getting paid for all of their hours. Also, the record keeping involved to document compliance is difficult. Therefore, it may be easier to use a lower hourly rate and pay employees for all hours on duty. If you need employees to work overtime, for out-of-town trips, special-event coverage, or any other reason, the time-and-one-half amount paid will be lower.

Matching Staff to the Call Load. Keep two things in mind while preparing a schedule for the service: when the calls occur and the number of calls. The same reports discussed for system-status management which listed the runs by time and day are also important for determining when to staff a vehicle. With system-status management, the emphasis is on *where* to place the vehicles. It's just as important to determine how many vehicles are needed. If there's a peak period for emergency and non-emergency runs, it may be necessary to add additional crews for prompt response time. Many services, therefore, add additional crews to handle peak loads. But the only way to accurately determine a service's special staffing needs is to prepare comprehensive reports on when and where ambulances are needed. Only then will there be enough information to make a valid decision.

The number of calls is also important. Even though the 24-hour shift has a number of advantages as previously discussed, there can be some serious disadvantages. A single crew can't be expected to respond on 20 separate ambulance calls during a 24-hour period and not experience fatigue, resulting in poor patient care. There's not a specific number of runs which a 24-hour team should be able to handle. There are many variables. Some of these include the ratio of emergencies to routines, the average length of the call, the times that the calls occur and the seriousness of the incidents. All of these affect the fatigue levels of EMTs and paramedics. A single crew might be able to handle 15 routine transfers without experiencing decreased energy levels. At the same time, two or three serious vehicle accidents may significantly decrease their ability to function adequately.

Reserve Production Capacity. The field of emergency medical transportation is unpredictable. Therefore, most of us have to provide a reserve pool of vehicles and personnel to meet unexpected demands. There are a number of ways to meet these demands.

Some services require off-duty personnel to carry pagers or to leave telephone numbers where they can be reached if extra help is needed. This is an effective way to ensure that experienced personnel are available to staff additional units. But it also decreases the individual's free time. Free time is important when on-duty shifts are long and stressful. If on-call is used, the staff should be paid a premium for being available and if called in, should receive additional time-and-a-half pay for their work.

A reserve program also provides additional staffing for a needed unit. These reserve personnel are not full-time employees, but are trained and able to staff vehicles. Continuing education, ride-along requirements and careful orientation are needed to make these people a valuable asset. Reserve employees are either volunteer or paid. Police departments have used this type of program for years with great success. This program also provides a pool from which to draw future employees.

A less frequently used approach is to cross train other personnel in the organization. Often, members of management have large amounts of street experience. Other personnel, including billing and secretarial staff can be trained to EMT levels to provide almost immediate production capacity if needed.

ULTIMATE LEGAL ACCOUNTABILITY

Legal accountability involves weeks of preparation, stress, sitting for hours on benches, waiting (only to be told the matter has been continued), badgering attorneys, dealing with impatient judges, not to mention spending thousands of dollars in legal fees and losing valuable time. And this is the best scenario—when you win. If you lose, you could fare worse: actual damages, punitive damages, the other party's legal fees, loss of credibility, reputation and possibly your job. Worse yet, you could be placed on probation or sent to jail if the violation is criminal in nature. *That's accountability!*

Whereas a great deal has been written about legal issues pertaining to prehospital care, little has been written about legal issues pertaining to EMS managers. There are two major areas of legal concern. These are legal issues that apply to any corporation, government or volunteer organization and issues that are specifically related to the operation of an ambulance service. Issues of general interest include compliance within general corporate law, tax matters, general liability, employment issues, compliance with statutory and legislative requirements for licensure, compliance with other regulatory matters such as OSHA, wages and zoning laws.

Issues specific to ambulance services include compliance with ambulance licensure law, medical malpractice, good-samaritan laws, compliance with Medicare and Medicaid reimbursement regulations, FCC, liability of first responders, who determines death, antitrust matters and compliance with state licensing-agency regulations.

DEALING WITH ATTORNEYS

The Service's Attorney. Developing a positive working relationship with the organization's attorney is fundamental to the success of the EMS manager. A trusting relationship is important because the attorney can be a positive influence with the board and community. In general, he can act as your sounding board. By discussing matters early you can avoid later heartache and expense. Don't skimp! Attorneys, however, are like auto mechanics. Find a good one who's

experienced in the type of problems you might have. You wouldn't
let a backyard mechanic work on a telemetry radio. So don't let a
general attorney represent the service in a malpractice case. A
competent attorney will not be offended if you suggest using a
specialist.

All Other Attorneys. Managers should be cautious of informal
discussions with other attorneys. This can backfire. In one case, an
attorney was reviewing records while talking with crew members
about a suit against a police officer involved in a traffic accident. The
attorney subsequently brought the ambulance service into the suit,
raising a malpractice issue.

From time to time, attorneys will request patient records. Before
disclosing any information, be sure to have a signed release from the
patient or a court order. Patients' medical records are otherwise
confidential. Services can charge attorneys for copies of patient
records. Some services have charged $50 for a record search.

Before responding to any outside legal request for information,
notify your service attorney about the request and tell him how you'd
like to respond. Screening responses through an attorney can avoid
costly errors. A motto to remember is, "When in doubt, contact the
service's attorney!"

C A S E   S T U D Y   # 8

Accountability

It's Monday morning. Joel, director of Goodwill EMS, is sitting at
his desk without the benefit of a cup of coffee. He's staring at his desk
piled with paperwork from the weekend, when the phone rings. The
mayor's office is calling. Fred, a top assistant to the mayor is irate.

"What's going on down there? I called over a week ago about a
complaint that some fool smashed an antique vase for no reason while
on a call at the Jones' house. The people are now threatening to sue
us for damages, and *nobody* seems to know what's going on. Are your
people incompetent or is everybody just 'out to lunch'? This is the
mayor's office. . . are you listening? I want an answer and I want it this
morning!"

Joel keeps his composure throughout and, after getting the
particulars of the incident, tells the mayor's aide that he'll get back to
him within the hour. As he puts the phone down he thinks, "Oh boy,
we're going to catch it now!"

"Damn," Joel says under his breath, realizing that the operations manager is on vacation. A moment of panic sweeps over him. He checks the service-inquiry log on the secretary's desk and breathes a sigh of relief. "Ah, there it is. February 17, Service Inquiry File Number 87–01. That means its the first complaint of the new year." He pulls the folder. All the information's there. The original inquiry from the mayor's office, the run report, the crew's written report and the summary of the disposition.

Joel walks into the mayor's office 27 minutes after Fred called. Fred looks up, visibly surprised to see him.

"Fred, I've reviewed the file you called about this morning and have the facts and a copy of all our records. According to our records, Mrs. Jones suffered a cardiac arrest last week. The unit had a response time of 3.2 minutes. When the crew arrived, the situation looked grave. The supplemental report written by the crew following your inquiry indicated that the housekeeper became hysterical when she discovered Mrs. Jones was not breathing. The vase you referred to was on the landing. We were doing CPR coming down the stairs and the housekeeper was trying to be helpful by moving it out of the way. She dropped it.

"Your original inquiry stated that Mrs. Jones' daughter was pleased with the service, but was unhappy that the $750 vase was broken. The supervisor verified the crew's supplemental report by calling the housekeeper and the police officer on the scene. These calls were made from the dispatch center on taped lines. If we need to document it further, tapes are available. Apparently, due to Mrs. Jones' illness, the daughter has not talked with the housekeeper."

Fred, impressed by such detail, momentarily softened then blustered, "Well that's all well and good, but how come I didn't get a response when I called?"

Joel broke into a broad grin as he said, "I'm glad you asked. According to the record, we received the original call from you on the 17th. The operations manager called with the information you requested at 1:30 p.m. on the 18th. According to the notes in the file I've copied for you, you were out to lunch and apparently didn't return his call. At 9:18 a.m. on the 19th he again unsuccessfully tried to reach you. He spoke with your secretary and relayed the information to her. She indicated that she would review it with you and that if any further action were required, she would be in touch. Fred, this is the only service inquiry EMS has had this year. But to avoid the confusion of missed messages in the future, how can we be assured that you get the information? By the way Fred, we saved Mrs. Jones' life."

The moral to this true case is this: be sure of your facts and be responsive. To do this make sure your internal tracking systems function and document the critical information. Startle people with your responsiveness to their inquiry.

■   ■   ■

Management of The Communications System and Understanding EMS Dispatching

Overview

Communications is the lifeline of an ambulance service, but it can be surrounded by a technical mystique that can be very intimidating to the uninitiated. EMS managers *must* have a working knowledge of the basics to be effective. Don't let the jargon of the technicians put you off. Once you get into it, you'll find it a simpler science than it looks from the outside.

EMS communications have increased in importance in the past several years as more and more services recognize the liability of poor systems, and the financial and service advantages of excellent systems. The priority dispatch system developed by Jeff Clawson, MD, has become the model by which services throughout the country are improving services. How well trained and motivated your communications people are, and how effective the *system* is they have to work with, is critical to your organization's ability to excel in general.

EMERGENCY AMBULANCE CALL

The most demanding responses upon personnel, equipment, system design, and financial resources are emergency assignments. These calls demand immediate life-saving action. Unfortunately, many services have built-in inefficiencies in the system. In order to streamline emergency responses, carefully review how your organization receives and handles each emergency call. A review of the chain of events which occur during an emergency will help to demonstrate the vital role communications plays. The order in which events occur in an emergency situation follows:

■ Chain of Events

1. The incident occurs.
2. The incident is discovered.
3. The incident is reported.
4. The report is processed by dispatchers.
5. The ambulance crew is dispatched.
6. The crew mans the vehicle, if they're not already in it.
7. The vehicle travels to the scene.
8. The vehicle arrives at the scene.
9. The patients are stabilized, treated and placed in the ambulance.
10. The ambulance leaves for the hospital.
11. The patients are transported to the hospital.
12. The ambulance arrives at the hospital.
13. The patients are unloaded, the crew completes their paperwork and the vehicle is readied for the next call.
14. The ambulance and crew announce their availability for another run.
15. The vehicle travels to post.
16. The vehicle arrives at post.

This list may be stating the obvious. However, anytime a system is evaluated and made more efficient, individual elements need to be broken down for evaluation. Let's say your objective for next year is to reduce the total time spent on a call by 25 percent. Which of the preceding steps could you effectively eliminate to reduce the time spent on a call? As a manager, you recognize that some of the time lags are beyond your control. It will be impossible to reduce the amount of time between steps 1 and 2, for example. Unless the National Guard patrols highways and local bars to discover incidents shortly after they occur, you would do well to concentrate your team's efforts in areas where a difference can be made.

Look at steps 2 through 6—from the time the incident is discovered to the moment just before the vehicle is en route to the scene. There are a number of things the EMS system can do to reduce these times. Strong community education outlining what to do in an emergency and development of an areawide 911 telephone system can significantly reduce this time. If you already have a 911 system, how efficient is it? Is it presently effective in saving time? Is it well advertised? By addressing these questions, you may be able to reduce time.

Steps 4 and 5 encompass call receiving and dispatching. The person who receives the call for help must be able to quickly notify the ambulance crew for an immediate response. In other words—*dispatch*. The dispatching system of many services is extremely weak, often deadly. No one is immune from problems and liabilities associated with dispatching. This was poignantly demonstrated in Dallas, Texas, in 1984, during a disastrous interaction between a call-screening nurse and a caller. Because the nurse focused on the caller's behavior, which included profanity, and not on the issue, she delayed the ambulance's dispatch and the caller's stepmother died. In 1987, calls to the 911 telephone system in Washington, D.C., were initially answered by a tape-recorded message. Dispatchers were reportedly careless and callous, much to the outrage of the media and general public. It's easy to see how an EMS system's hard-earned credibility can be destroyed in just moments by such events.

CALL SCREENING VS. PRIORITY DISPATCHING

Part of the issue here involves recognition of emergency medical dispatch (EMD) as a vital part of the emergency process. Some confusion has been raised in the industry over two terms: call screening and priority dispatching.

Call screening is when a dispatcher, paramedic or nurse answers emergency telephone calls to screen out those that are frivolous or to determine what emergency response should be sent. Depending on the system, this may include differentiating between BLS and ALS needs. In all ALS systems, it may mean deciding if the paramedics should use lights and sirens or whether or not to send first responders at all. Some places allow the person taking the call to assess over the telephone whether or not a response is indicated (a practice regarded as a tremendous risk).

Priority dispatching encompasses more than call screening. Here, the caller is asked set questions to help determine how that situation fits a preset response configuration. The concept also includes pre-arrival telephone first-aid instructions—a wonderful stop-gap measure for critical situations as well as a highly regarded local public-relations tool–when done right.

The initial system for priority dispatching was developed by Jeff J. Clawson, M.D., for use by Utah's Salt Lake City Fire Department. With this type of system, mistakes regarding patient care are avoided. Each system using priority dispatch customizes appropriate responses to meet the varying needs of patients. Even volunteer EMS systems can organize their priorities to vary the response sent, instead of sending everyone with lights flashing and sirens blaring—a practice clearly frought with risks.

Many small services don't use either call screening or priority dispatch. If callers request emergency, they get emergency. There's generally one level of care provided. This system may work well for a smaller service, but it can expose a community to unnecessary emergency traffic and the hazards associated with it. Some situations may require listing assignments according to their priority. Decisions of this nature should be made with the help of established written protocols that are approved by the local medical community. If no system is in place, the manager creates liability and expects dispatchers to make decisions without the necessary authority, direction or training.

EMS call-handling and dispatch procedures must be clearly written to cover most situations that may be encountered. Without such procedures and the necessary training, the EMS provider, communications center and communications personnel may be liable for mistakes.

Problems can arise anytime the call handler or dispatcher is required to make decisions concerning any one of the following:

What information is needed from the caller?
What instructions should be given to the caller?
Whether or not to send an ALS or BLS unit, or both.
Whether or not to send a first responder.
Whether or not to send multiple EMS units.
Whether or not to notify or request other agencies or services.
Where the call should be placed in queue.

The decision process should be well defined and in writing. This will eliminate the possibility of making a wrong decision which could result in harm to a patient or legal liablility to an EMS system.

SYSTEM-STATUS MANAGEMENT

In the past few years, system-status management has become a common term in EMS. Every service uses system-status management in some form, whether in the dispatcher's head, on paper or in the computer. System-status management is simply the strategy used for placement of ambulances and crews based on expected call volumes and locations. It's used to reduce response times. In its most sophisticated form, it uses computers and other technologies. In its simplest form, it calls for placing the one available unit in a centralized location. All services can benefit by formalizing the process of strategic unit deployment.

Let's look at the simplest case again. There is one vehicle. The service provides emergency response for an entire county. You decide to place that ambulance right in the middle of the county. That's the fairest way to do it. Responses can be made to all four corners of the county in the same amount of time, right? Wrong! Geography is not your only consideration. Where do most of the people live? Where do most calls usually occur?

There is a medium-sized town in the north-central part of the county. Most of the people live in this town. What does that say? You decide to move your ambulance's post to the southern edge of the town. You're getting closer. That's the idea behind system-status management. But is that area really in the center of the requests for emergency help? While geography and population influence the decision, you must also determine any patterns to the locations of emergency incidents. Maybe most of the emergency responses are directed toward an interstate at the southern edge of the county or toward a group of taverns on the western county line. These emergency assignments should be taken into consideration when placing ambulances. The only way to determine the best placement is to plot on a map (by hand or computer simulation), the locations of emergency calls over a period of time.

One way to determine emergency response locations is to use colored pins on a large map. Randomly select a period of time, with enough emergency calls, to establish a pattern. Place a pin for each emergency call location. Different colored pins can be used to distinguish different types of calls or various times of the day. After a few hundred pins a pattern may develop. By carefully identifying the areas with higher concentrations of pins (calls), you can then make an intelligent decision about vehicle placement. You can also back up your decision to others by showing them the map.

Is that all there is to system-status management? No, but for many services this would be an improvement over what they have. What other variables need to be considered? Many larger systems using system-status management base pin placement on days of the week and hours of the day. Where do the ambulances need to be placed at 10 a.m. on Tuesdays for example? Not only is location considered, but also the number of crews needed. To determine this, many maps are pinned—one map for each hour of each day of each week. Other variables can be considered—season of the year, weather, special activities and other considerations may influence the locations of emergencies. There may be something to the idea that more emergencies occur during a full moon. Sophisticated system-status management could help to prove or disprove it. It's easy to see why some of the larger services, with thousands of monthly calls, resort to computer assistance to help determine the stationing possibilities for their crews. Complete system-status management entails moving the post locations of the different crews, sometimes on an hourly basis to achieve the shortest possible response times.

The crucial point in this section is not necessarily how much of the system-status management process is used, but that there is some rationale and validation of why and where ambulance resources are placed. Good management of the system will help to reduce response times as well as the total time a crew will be tied up with a particular call.

COMMUNICATIONS PERSONNEL TRAINING

Training for EMS dispatchers is of the utmost importance. The lives of many rest in the hands of a few. The stress a dispatcher feels can be likened to the stress felt by an air-traffic controller. The support and training for these people is an often overlooked necessity. "If you can't make it in the field, you can always be a dispatcher" is a dangerous philosophy. Dispatchers should be screened and trained to high levels of proficiency. The workings of the entire system depend on them. They can make the most difficult situations run smoothly or turn routine into chaos. The system's manager must provide his dispatchers with the proper tools to do their job well. Whenever possible, they should be medically trained. They should have guidelines for normal operations as well as special procedures for system overloads. Define their role for them in disaster situations and develop written procedures.

Dispatchers are the first contact between the service and the patient or his family. How a call is handled often determines how well the call will proceed from that point. That in turn influences the patient's or family's opinion about the service provided. Dispatchers are also public-relations officers, those polite and concerned professionals who will get help for those in need. They also relay basic, and many times lifesaving, emergency medical-care instructions over the phone for bystanders to perform until help arrives.

Good dispatchers must be able to calm the hysterical, interview the non-listening, to get information to pass on to demanding and oftentimes unforgiving crews. If you detect admiration for the oft forgotten and unsung heroes of EMS, you're right!

The two primary tools of a dispatcher are the telephone and the radio. Most calls for help will be received by phone. Most ambulances are dispatched by radio. To be effective, both tools require specific skills and procedures. Specific procedures for obtaining information from a caller and using the radios are outlined in many courses designed for communications personnel. It's well worth the time and expense to provide this available training for the dispatcher.

QUESTIONS FOR THE EVALUATION OF AN EMS COMMUNICATIONS CENTER

Having an efficient dispatcher and good procedures for system-status management can decrease the length of calls, especially response time to an emergency site. To evaluate your dispatch system, ask yourself these questions:

1. Have all communications personnel been trained (communications course, system-status management, EMT or EMT-P and disaster procedures)?
2. Is pay for your communications personnel equal to, or greater than, the field personnel?
3. Are routine and emergency procedures written down?
4. Is an ambulance dispatched within 45 seconds of receiving an emergency call?
5. Are all emergency and non-emergency calls dispatched from the same location?
6. Is the dispatch center tied into 911 telephone service?
7. Is system-status management an integral part of the system?
8. Do your dispatchers have immediate communication capabilities with other public-safety officials (fire and law-enforcement agencies)?
9. Does the dispatch center have emergency-power capability?
10. Are all times *accurately* documented?
11. Are radio and telephone conversations recorded on an instant-recall and semi-permanent basis?
12. Is a log kept of all calls (transport and non-transport)?
13. Can your dispatchers identify the location and status of all ambulances at all times?
14. Do they give telephone emergency-care instructions if approved and appropriate?
15. Are your dispatchers able to control telephone conversations with callers?
16. Are all calls answered on the first or second ring?
17. Do communications personnel have a resource book for requesting specialized assistance (cranes, tow trucks, divers, radioactive monitors, hazardous materials experts, etc.)?
18. Do you have an effective local emergency-management plan? Are your dispatchers trained to use it?

19. Is priority dispatch used and well-defined by protocols?
20. Do your dispatchers have field experience?
21. Are they allowed to perform their primary function? Have inappropriate extra jobs been eliminated from their work load?
22. Are your dispatchers given adequate equipment to do their jobs well (telephones, radios, time clocks, recorders, maps, and so on)?
23. Are dispatchers familiar with local geography and traffic patterns?

These are only some of the questions to ask. If the answer is yes to each of the above questions, you have a very good system, indeed. Most managers will be able to identify some weaknesses, but that's the purpose of the questions. Set up an action plan to correct them. Keep in mind the object is to reduce delays and minimize mistakes. A list and description of communications and other dispatch equipment is included in the Communications Hardware section of this book.

IMPROVING SYSTEM EFFICIENCY

Although the following correlates with our earlier discussion on training, we feel it important to combine it here with the chain of events in an emergency ambulance call (see the listing earlier in this section). Response times to the scene *can* be safely reduced through training as the following discussion of "chain of events" steps 6 through 16 will illustrate. Steps 6 through 8 in the emergency-call chain of events encompass the response of the emergency vehicle and crew. As discussed earlier, some reduction in response time can take place in these steps. But the manager must be careful to emphasize the right step. It's OK to encourage time reductions in step 6, manning the vehicle, but caution should be used in emphasizing reduction of travel time to the scene, step 7. Some services penalize their crews if they don't man their vehicles within a minute's notice. Penalties are not recommended. Instead, consider developing healthy competition between crews followed by positive reinforcement. Keep track of the various times it takes each crew to man its vehicle for emergency calls. Post the times, and praise the quicker teams. Peer pressure will probably be enough stimulus for quicker responses. Some services have their dispatchers radio a second alert when the crew hasn't staffed its vehicle within one minute. They might say "Medic-3, respond to 6th and Main, man down, priority one, SECOND ALERT." This not only notifies the crew that its response is slow, but everyone else in the system hears it as well. No one likes to be singled out for poor effort. This is an effective way to reduce response times.

There's only one appropriate way to increase response time in step 7—TRAINING. A heavy foot on the gas pedal is dangerous and is apt to result in no response. Safe driving should be a primary concern for EMS managers. Speed is not professional! The fascination with speed and the thrill of tearing down city streets at 80 mph no longer have a place in this profession. EMS vehicles don't have carte blanche to ignore the safety of others. The courts of law have also made that clear by rendering judgments against emergency personnel for speeding even on emergency calls. Most liability cases against EMS services don't stem from patient care, but are the result of traffic accidents involving vehicles. The opinions and attitudes of the staff may have to be modified to accept these ideas. Specific guidelines for emergency responses must be established and enforced. Safe arrival at the scene far outweighs any benefit gained by careening through the community at high speed.

Response times to the scene can be safely reduced through training. Familiarity with the geography and traffic-flow patterns are the most important. Selection of the proper route to the scene will effectively and safely reduce the time it takes to get there. Staying on main thoroughfares and avoiding known-to-be congested areas at particular times of the day make for a smoother and quicker response. The dispatcher can assist by notifying the crew of any abnormal congestion, road construction or other traffic problem.

Step 9, time spent at the scene, generally accounts for the largest block of time spent on an emergency ambulance call. This is appropriate for patient extrication, examination, treatment and stabilization. This is what paramedics are trained for. Even so, this should be time well-spent, not wasted, especially for critical-trauma victims. The clock on the golden hour starts ticking when the injury occurs, not when the ambulance arrives. For the critical-trauma patient, only lifesaving procedures should be attempted at the scene (for example, establishing an airway, controlling severe hemorrhage and stabilizing the victim). Any other ALS procedures should be done en route to the hospital. This is directly opposed to the treatment of the medical case, such as heart attack, where studies show that initial treatment at the scene is more important than immediate transport. Your system should have medical protocols to account for both of these important strategies.

How can scene time be reduced? Train–practice–train–practice–train.... Studies have shown that in most critical situations a well-organized ALS team shouldn't be on the scene more than 12 to 14 minutes. This provides ample time for diagnosis and treatment. If each paramedic is expert, the team will need less time to provide the best possible care. We need to emphasize EXPERT, not just proficient.

Now for step 11. The same philosophy of not making up time with speed applies here as well. We've all snickered at "another" ambulance service communicating information about a patient with a broken toe, while in the background its siren's wailing away. But it's not so funny when we hear the siren during a report about a patient with acute chest pain. And maybe it's not "another" service that's being monitored. There are few true life-threatening emergencies needing red lights and sirens to a hospital. There are even fewer situations for which ALS services should transport patients in the emergency mode. The possible time saved can be negated by the extra physical and emotional trauma the patient suffers by the high stress of emergency transport. Design your system so that true life-threatening emergencies can be identified and the majority of patient transports handled in a cautious non-emergency fashion.

Once crew members deliver the patient to the hospital and give their patient report, their primary responsibility to that patient is fulfilled. It's important that they now prepare themselves for the next call. Generally, one crew member cleans and restocks the ambulance while the other completes all necessary paperwork. Every effort should be made to reservice the vehicle as quickly as possible. You don't know when the next emergency, or batch of emergencies, will occur. Reducing down time at the hospital increases your service's resource availability to handle all of the calls.

One service had an average hospital down time of 43 minutes. Management couldn't understand why ambulances weren't available to meet their demands. It's obvious that if crews are unavailable for an hour after each run, a lot of their resources are going to waste. Other services have *average* hospital down times of eight to 12 minutes.

So now you mandate that crews spend no more than 15 minutes at the hospital. Wait a minute. It may not be that the crews are wasting time. It may well be that the system still has some holes in it. Has the service provided extra equipment at the hospital or in the vehicles, or is the crew having to wait for the backboard, anti-shock trousers, or traction splint? Have procedures been worked out with the hospital so the crew can deliver their patient to the emergency room, or are they having to take the patient back to the X-ray department or to a floor? Do they have to get all of the patient information at the hospital, even if it means waiting for family members to arrive? Each situation is different. There may be a number of reasons for time spent at the hospital. If you've measured hospital time and think it should be reduced, look at what's taking the time. Talk to your crews and appropriate hospital personnel before developing policies to effect improvement of the turn-around time. It's also important your crews ready themselves and their equipment even if they're at the hospital waiting for equipment or information. As soon as the vehicle is ready to respond to a call, the crew should notify dispatch that they're available and can respond from the hospital if a call comes in.

A final point to help improve your system's efficiency. Reduce your crews' extra activities when they're not on an assigned call. Crews should not be assigned errands or be allowed to run personal errands. Both can interfere with a fast response to an emergency call. Cruising, errand-running, not only wastes gas and increases wear and tear on the vehicle, but decreases your service's dependable response time. It's difficult for dispatchers and supervisors to keep track of rolling vehicles. So avoid errant errands.

C A S E   S T U D Y   # 9

Improving System Efficiency

Tom Jones is EMS director of the Cornertown Fire Department. He's been with the fire department for eight years and has been EMS director for the past three years.

The fire chief has just returned from a finance committee meeting with the city council. His face is ashen, and he looks exhausted. The news isn't good!

"Tom, we've got to increase our efficiency. Our EMS call volume is increasing and our response times are barely in compliance with the 90 percent within eight minutes. The committee won't increase our budget. If anything, it'd like to see it reduced. The finance committee couldn't be dissuaded. I tried my best."

Tom has anticipated this committee action as the city had been in financial difficulty ever since the nearby steel plant closed down. But he'd never seen the chief look so upset before, and that bothered him. Reducing service standards wasn't an option. He and the chief both agreed on that.

Tom had developed an informal crisis council—a casual group of medics and supervisors which he convened from time to time to help him brainstorm and evaluate options for particularly difficult issues. The group usually met over a few beers in his living room. Sometimes they had helped him to see another side of an issue. Often they helped him understand the impact of a particular course of action. Over the years, most were able to detach themselves from their own opinions and look at any particular situation objectively. Tom thought this would be a good time to ask them to help him "think it out."

In less than half an hour the group brainstormed 17 ideas. They didn't evaluate any one idea, but instead just listed them. The initial list of ideas was wide ranging. Some of the ideas were great. Some not so workable. Tom was careful at this point not to evaluate or criticize any of the initial ideas.

The team then grouped the ideas by categories and placed the remaining list of ideas in priority for detailed discussion. As the discussion unfolded, Tom was impressed with the medics' concerns for quality of service rather than their own interests. They all agreed three steps could be taken to provide better service with the same resources.

Bill brought up that in the last month seven calls were missed because a unit had broken down and the crew was re-stocking a spare unit. The equipment was locked in the storeroom so the crew spent over an hour stripping the out-of-service vehicle's gear and placing it on the spare unit. It seemed to make more sense to keep all the units stocked and locked to make such a transition easy.

"That's a super idea," said Tom. The group seemed encouraged by his approval.

Another medic said, "Tom, we seem to get busy right around shift change. That creates additional overtime when we get held over, not to mention messing up our day off. What about staggering some of the shift change times to help out?"

"We've read about flexible staffing in *jems* but we've never really analyzed what the operational and economic considerations would be here," one of the supervisors said. "Operationally it would mean a central or regional relief system and a loss of permanent stations, but it could give us as much as 20 percent more productivity."

Bill was skeptical about flexible staffing, listing several negative aspects. Tom was afraid that the process might break down.

"Bill, we've looked at some of the concerns about flexible staffing," Tom said. "Now let's look at a few positive considerations."

Sam offered that a variety of shifts would be appreciated by some of the crew members going to school.

"I'd much rather work a bit harder but fewer days, which is possible with flex-staffing," another group member added.

Tom added, "If we do go to a flex-staff program, we can consolidate some of our training positions and use them as a last-out unit in the system. It's not often that we get to a last-out status which would enable them to conduct most of their training functions without interruption."

Tom looked at his watch and was surprised to see it was past midnight. The group had become so involved that they had all lost track of time. To sum up their evening's work, Tom said, "Each of these ideas could be tough to implement. It'll take all of us working together if its going to work. Why don't we each think about what would be involved in implementing these ideas and get together next week? I'll ask the chief if he would stop by one evening so we can review our plan with him."

■   ■   ■

COMMUNICATIONS HARDWARE AND SYSTEMS

The EMS manager wears many hats. One of those is that of the communications expert. Let's face it, good radio communication equipment is vital in order to provide high-quality patient-care services. Advancements in medical communications have helped improve prehospital medical care in the last decade and a half. Managers who understand their service's needs can then make intelligent decisions regarding an appropriate communications system. Whether the system is centralized or decentralized, sophisticated or unsophisticated, basic elements are necessary for appropriate communications. The concept is simple. Implementing it is not.

What are the components of an EMS communications system? Not the pieces of equipment. That comes later. What does the system need in the way of communications? Look at Figure 4.6. This diagram demonstrates the need for two-way communication between different agencies and their personnel.

The EMS system has specialized needs, but also interconnects with existing systems in the region. The trend today, with tightened budgets and increased expectations for the quality of service, is toward consolidating dispatch centers. A consolidated or cooperative dispatch center pools a number of participating services—their equipment, facilities, personnel, and of course, funding. Representatives for all of the participating jurisdictions determine the cooperative's operation and procedures. This works well in many areas where the various departments can't easily fund their own dispatch facilities. It also promotes cooperation and coordination among the various services.

■ Equipment needs of the medical communications center

Radios. Provide radios to communicate with ambulances and other services. These should be as powerful as possible and connect to an antenna high enough to cover the region served (UHF and/or VHF).

Backup radio. A method of providing backup communications should the main radio fail.

Paging facilities. Facilities to notify off-duty and on-call crews.

Radio frequencies.

> *Communications.* This is the service's own frequency. Some may use the hospital frequency. This communication frequency can either be VHF or UHV (med 9 or 10).

Figure 4.6   Radio Communications

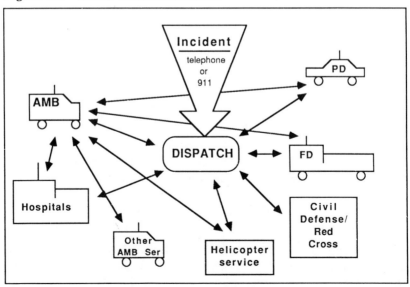

Public-safety communications to fire or law enforcement. The communications center should be able to contact other public safety services for backup assistance or information. Ideally, this should be done by radio, so that mobile units can be contacted. At least a dedicated telephone should be available.

Hospital communications. It may be necessary for communications personnel to talk directly to hospitals, especially in disaster situations.

*Communications to other ambulances and agencies.*Communications personnel may be called upon to coordinate activities with other services, especially in disaster situations. Communications capabilities with civil defense, other ambulance services and helicopter services are among the possibilities.

Telephones. Provide adequate telephones and incoming lines so that no one receives a busy signal when calling for help. The only time the system should be overloaded is during a disaster or other unusual situation. Consider an unlisted private line for emergency communication to the dispatch center or so that the center can contact other public agencies without interfering with incoming calls.

Scanner. It's good practice for dispatchers to be aware of the activities of other public safety agencies. This may forewarn them of the possible need of ambulance dispatch. A good scanner will give dispatch a wealth of information on what's going on in the region.

Weather monitor. Many civil defense agencies provide area resources with alert monitors. This is valuable during hazardous weather conditions.

Time recorder. Provide a way to accurately record time. Whether by clock or computer, consistently document time.

Voice recorder. Recording radio and phone conversations is important. Future legal questions and the promotion of service efficiency are good reasons for documenting these conversations by a voice recorder.

Emergency power. In case of a power blackout, it's necessary to be able to maintain the basic functions of your dispatch center. This is apt to be a time of increased demand on your service.

■ Communications needs for the vehicle

Mobile radios. Multifrequency radio. VHF for hospital frequency, law enforcement and fire agencies. An encoder which looks like a telephone dial is needed. This is used to open communication with hospital radios so hospital personnel can hear the message. The FCC has also allocated frequencies on the UHF band for emergency medical services. If these med channels are going to be used, a separate UHF radio is required, with some or all of the med-channel frequencies installed. (More about UHF later in this section.)

Rear control. The rear headset or handset in the patient compartment is an extension of the radio. This allows the attendant to talk to the hospital and report on the patient's condition. It also allows the driver to pay attention to his driving instead of trying to relay radio communications.

Hand-held radio. The walkie-talkie radio should be given to at least one crew member. This enables the dispatcher to contact the crew, even when they're out of their rig. Pagers can also be used, but they're not as effective for field technicians, because they can't be used to call for help while the technicians are outside of their vehicle.

Portable med-radio. This radio differs from the hand-held radio in that it's primarily used to relay patient information and telemetry from the scene. It's a UHF radio, equipped with the appropriate med channels which can be received by the hospital. Although telemetry is sometimes transmitted over phone lines, eliminating the need for this radio, many victims are not conveniently located next to a phone.

Vehicular repeater (possible need). If your service area is large or if the area's geography makes radio transmission from lower-powered portable med radios to the hospital difficult, then a repeater may be necessary. The vehicular repeater takes the weak signal from the portable med radio, amplifies it to the power level of the vehicle's mobile radio, and re-transmits it to the hospital receiver.

■ Alerting crew members

Once a call is received, there must be a way to alert the crew. Telephones, pagers, sirens and radios are only some of the methods used. When selecting the best method for your service, keep in mind that communication is most efficient when it's two-way. Dispatchers need feedback to assure them that the crew heard the call and is en route. The crew members, on the other hand, will be more comfortable if they can ask specific questions about the location or type of call. Therefore, these considerations eliminate many of the possible methods of alerting the unit. A telephone provides two-way communication, but what if the crews are in the ambulance?

Pagers and radios are the most effective means of dispatch. In case of power failure, emergency electric power can easily be provided. An auxiliary radio (hand-held or mobile) can be used if the main base-station radio fails. Portable radios and pagers keep dispatchers in contact with the crews even when they're outside their vehicles. And finally, be sure to provide uniformity in dispatch. Systems which use multiple methods of unit notification are prone to confusion and mistakes.

■ Unit en route and at the scene

An ambulance responding to a call has its own communications needs. The EMTs and paramedics need to be able to communicate with the communications center, but they may also need to talk to other public-safety agencies and first responders. Minimum capability should include the ability to communicate with local law-enforcement officials, fire departments, other ambulance services, first responders, the communications center and hospitals. By being able to talk to law-enforcement personnel, field personnel can get help in finding difficult locations and assistance when confronted by a violent situation or crime scene. Fire departments are often called upon to assist with rescue or extrication, and good coordination between on-the-scene crews is a must. Use first responders, for the responding crew should be able to talk to these trained personnel, to give instructions and to learn more about the patient's situation prior to arrival.

Before installing and using the frequencies licensed to other services, it's necessary to obtain permission and formulate procedures for their use.

■ At the scene and en route to the hospital

Equipment needs for ambulance vehicles also apply here, with emphasis on communication with the hospital. In ALS services, communication with the medical-control physician is essential. Direct radio contact is usually via UHF med channels. The advantage of using UHF is that the system is designed for duplex transmission. The best way to understand duplex is to think of the telephone. Both people on the telephone can talk and be heard at the same time. This is also true of duplex. It takes two separate frequencies to provide this communication—one for transmission and one for receiving. A second means for hospital communication is also often available with a VHF radio, which is normally a simplex system. Many services use VHF transmissions for those routine calls which don't require advanced procedures and UHF for direct contact with a physician. Many hospitals don't have UHF capability. Therefore, VHF radio communication is the only way to deliver patient information or receive medical-control orders. Hospital emergency departments should have a direct unlisted phone line. This enables field medics to use a telephone from the patient's location, when available, and not tie up the radio.

Telemetry is also a concern for ALS ambulance providers. Telemetry is the radio transmission of biomedical information, usually the patient's electrocardiogram, to a receiving hospital. This enables a physician to make a more specific diagnosis and provide proper orders to the paramedics. EKG patterns can be relayed to the hospital either by radio (almost always UHF) or by direct phone line. The hospital must have the proper de-modulating equipment to transform the signal into an EKG tracing.

Most progressive systems are moving away from telemetry and are depending on verbal descriptions of both the EKG strip and the patient's physical description. Many physicians believe that this is as reliable as, and more effective than, telemetry. Telemetry equipment is delicate and prone to breakage—despite good maintenance.

■ Hospital communications equipment

Before investing in new communications equipment, be sure it's compatible with the hospital system. It would do no good to install UHF equipment to communicate with an emergency room if that hospital's emergency room has no way to receive the signal. The same is true with telemetry. Installation of a telemetry system is a joint effort and must be planned carefully.

A hospital's communications equipment will usually include the following:

VHF radio. A majority of ambulance services only have VHF radio capability. The radio, or a remote extension, should be in the emergency department. Otherwise, direct communication with the emergency-room staff becomes difficult.

UHF radio. The trend in EMS communications is to use UHF med channels. The selected channels must be coordinated with the local ALS EMS services.

Demodulator. This equipment decodes impulses from the UHF radio or telephone line into signals that can be displayed on an EKG monitor and recorded on an EKG tracing.

Private unlisted phone line. This phone line to the emergency department can be used in lieu of the radio for both patient information and EKG transmission.

Recorder. It's a good idea for the hospital to record verbal and telemetric radio communications. This provides a good training aid for hospital and field personnel and can be used to determine the adequacy of treatment and procedures.

The trend in the industry is to get away from the vehicle system, with all its unrelated radio traffic, and toward UHF, which is strictly limited to EMS. The Federal Communication Commission (FCC) is the regulatory agency which governs all radio operations in the United States. The FCC allocates frequencies, systems, issues licenses and establishes power limitations. To help coordinate medical communications, in 1974 the FCC allocated new frequencies for EMS. The new FCC ruling provides specific frequencies for communication among ambulances, hospitals and communications centers, with separate higher-powered frequencies for portable radios. It also makes it possible to handle multiple incidents on different frequencies without conflict.

These new rules have established nation wide uniformity since the same channels are used throughout the country. It requires close coordination among EMS systems located in the same region. All types of EMS communications, including telemetry, are now being encouraged to use the 450-470 megahertz (MHz) UHF frequency band. All locations include two frequency pairs (462.950/467.950 and 462.975/467.975). These are considered the dispatch channels. The diagram below lists currently available frequencies and their primary and secondary roles as determined by the FCC. In addition, the FCC has designated four frequencies in the 458 MHz band for transmission from portable units to associated mobile units (repeating).

Also, new equipment in the 800MHz band is being licensed for EMS use and should be considered in congested urban areas.

The objective of the EMS communications system is to minimize time between the onset of the accident or illness and the rendering of emergency medical care. As discussed earlier, the communications system can be divided into four components: the initial call for help, the communications center, the ambulance and paramedic communications and the hospital communications.

While it's impossible to discuss all options and system configurations availble to EMS communications, it's important to emphasize that EMS managers have a basic knowledge of communications. Appendix A is a glossary that should help decipher the many complex terms used in the communications industry.

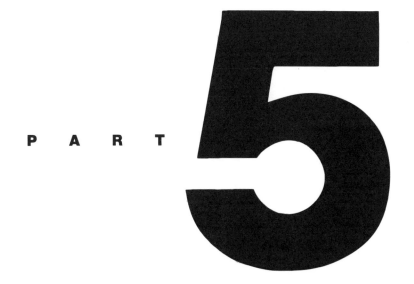

P A R T

Working With Other Teams— Groups That Affect Success

Why
We're Here

Overview

The primary objecive of any EMS organization is to
provide patient care. But this goal is often clouded or lost
during day-to-day operations or pressing concerns with
equipment, finance and personnel. The patient is the
consumer in our marketplace, and service our focus. Service
begins when the phone rings in dispatch requesting a
response, and continues for several weeks after the patient
has been transferred. Along the way, there are several places
where service can break down creating dissatisfied customers.
Some of you reading this may have trouble considering
patients as clients. EMS is a service business. There is a clear
distinction between regarding patients as clients and
regarding patients as victims. In this section we will examine
some of those areas that may require an extra effort in order
to prevent negative outcomes. We'll also look at the external
groups that interact with the delivery of patient care.

VIEWING THE PATIENT AS CLIENT

The patient's plea for personalized care is one of the most widely expressed criticisms of medical care today. This is more urgent to many health-care leaders than even the rising cost of care. When the two are linked together (high cost for ineffective, impersonal care), the result leaves a bitter aftertaste. Part of the team-building concept is developing each player's sensitivity to human needs—those of warmth and kindness and to help your staff to understand that personal attention to each client and his family plays an important part in retaining and increasing your service's image. Public or private, clients are the only reason organizations exist.

Law suits are on the increase. Patients and their family members have raised their voices not only in the service's offices, but in courts as well. Clients expect more from their emergency medical service and are quick to report negative experiences. In many cases clients aren't complaining about equipment quality or medical technology. Their complaints, instead, focus on the quality of personal caring they have—or haven't—received. It takes but a few caring words and quiet moments to convey you care.

To ensure client's rights are emphasized and respected, assess your team's level of professional integrity. How often do you find staff members talking *at* someone, rather than *with* someone? Is this the practice in the back of your units? Is your staff sharing *with* the client and family, or do your consumers listen to stories of the crew's last run, wondering what will be said of them after they're transported? Is your crew careful about what they say within earshot of the client? Is their discussion about the stupid mistakes the first responders made, or that maybe they should have called for a helicopter transport because the patient was critical? These are just a few examples of communications that violate the client's rights to confidentiality. Unfortunately, the back of the ambulance is not a vacuum, and the crews' words and actions will be remembered by the client.

Another aspect affecting the client's right to quality care is the team's collaborative effort. How well do team members work together? Is there harmony and continuity as the patient progresses through each phase of the health-care system? Developing smooth working relationships by defining each member's role and identifying where these roles overlap is the manager's responsibility to both staff and client. Establishing a working relationship among these interacting groups will alleviate disorganization, fragmentation of care and turf games as well as increase communication. Remember, patient care is the reason for each group's involvement, and that theme must remain foremost in everyone's mind at *all* times.

Players At
The Scene

Overview

All services run into occasional problems with other groups at the scene of an emergency. The key is to keep these differences *minor*. Remember, the patient doesn't care whose territory is being invaded, or whose feelings are being hurt. You owe to the patient the best possible service your community can provide, even if you have to swallow your pride sometimes. The street or a home is not the place for confrontations. You're not doing your job if you've allowed your field personnel to go out on a call without having already clearly defined their role in relationship with all the other groups they must work with.

Patient outcome will be improved the better the teams at the scene work together. Of critical importance is the first responders. This has been frequently demonstrated by communities with successful citizen CPR and first-responder programs. An added benefit, of course, is the good-will that can be created when your organization is active in training and organizing these programs.

FIRST RESPONDERS

Collaboration with a first-responder program must become part of your health-care service. The easiest approach is to personally sponsor a first-responder course, using staff, vehicles and equipment for the training. This will assist in external team building and construct bridges for effective communication. It will also help your staff take charge on emergency scenes.

In addition to organized public safety and volunteer first responders, consider citizen involvement. Programs like CPR NOW! in Seattle and Kansas City have had dramatic results. For example, in Kansas City, with the support of the Kansas City Royals baseball team, over 100,000 citizens were trained in CPR in less than two years. Ambulance officials have credited Kansas City's high cardiac-arrest survival rate to early citizen CPR intervention. A by-product has been an improved relationship with co-sponsoring agencies and a dramatically increased public image for the service.

All of this happened because someone involved in EMS persuaded the team's owner that their support was important. If you're thinking, "Well, Kansas City is a big town. We don't have those kinds of resources," don't! The scope of the CPR NOW! project was just as overwhelming for its creators as your project ideas may seem to you. The point is that with creative leadership much can be accomplished. What are you going to do?

SUPPORT TEAMS

It's a given that cooperation with all public safety personnel is essential in order to have the best possible emergency medical service for the patient. What is not well understood is how the EMS manager goes about establishing such cooperation when politics is not conducive to such and you're not sure who's in charge. Despite these obstacles, the manager is responsible for addressing these issues with his colleagues in order to avoid field personnel from working together with different authority and role expectations. The interaction between public-safety officials and EMS personnel must be predetermined in order to afford a smooth working area for the delivery of patient care. Each team needs to be recognized for the unique skill and talent they bring to patient care. It's important to realize that no single agency can perform the task without the complementing strengths of the other agencies.

HELICOPTER INTERVENTION AT THE SCENE

The use of aeromedical transport for prehospital care is becoming increasingly common. Helicopters offer a level of care and transport that can significantly increase the survival rates of critically ill or injured patients. They often provide personnel trained in advanced life-support care and equipment of benefit in those instances when time is crucial, when geography prohibits easy ground access and in multiple-patient incidents.

It's important that your employees know where these services are, how and when to activate an assist reponse from them and how to secure a safe landing area. Anytime a helicopter is brought to the scene, safety must be of primary concern. Preparation for those at the scene and of the landing area must be done quickly. Make sure your crews are well-versed in safety in order to transfer the patient without undue hazard.

Typically, a helicopter program provides training and literature for EMS providers. Your staff should be exposed to this information. Again, by establishing relationships with other prehospital groups, you'll enhance the effectiveness of *your* service.

The decision to call for air support should be preceded by company policy endorsed by the crew. They need to be familiar with helicopter response times, and use those time variables wisely when making decisions. For example, it wouldn't be appropriate to wait 20 minutes for a helicopter if the patient is ready for transport and the receiving hospital is only 10 away minutes by ground.

Other
Care Providers

Overview

In addition to the groups mentioned in the preceding sections, EMS services will have to deal with physicians who intervene at the scene, and physicians who order transportation from their private offices. Some services also will have to provide transportation from or to hospitals and nursing homes.

The progressive EMS manager will plan for these interactions to occur in as positive a way as possible. There are lots of opportunities in these settings for things to turn sour, but there are also opportunities to make a good impression.

One aspect of your job is to present your service in the best light possible to the medical community at large. There will always be physicians and other organizations who won't fully appreciate your service's role as a medical provider. Don't give them a foothold for dissent.

PHYSICIAN INTERVENTION

Planning for the likelihood of a physician at the scene includes establishing a written policy, endorsed by the medical director, the local health-department director or the medical society. It should include a statement or form that is available for the on-scene physician to sign, indicating that he assumes full responsibility for the patient and the patient's care. Many services have incorporated this form, as well as a patient refusal form, on the back of their run report. Local policy may require that the physician establish communication with your on-line medical director and accompany the patient to the receiving hospital.

CALLS TO PHYSICIANS' OFFICES

Requests to transfer patients from physicians' offices should be viewed as an opportunity to demonstrate your service's professionalism and performance while providing patient care. The private physician may have orders for you to follow, and they should be accommodated as long as the orders don't interfere with medical protocols. Any conflicting orders are to be resolved with the physician or the on-line medical-control physician prior to transport. Realize that this is often a stressful interaction for the physician. Psychologically, it's difficult for some physicians to admit they need help to save a person's life. Particularly when the medics are "such young whippersnappers" and are treading on the physician's home turf. No matter how distasteful such attitudes may be, medics must be aware they exist, and that it's wise for them to placate the physician.

Physicians who negate the role EMS plays in providing patient care generally have had a bad experience with over-zealous crews, or have not had the opportunity to personally participate in any phase of the EMS system. Prejudging them as opponents will only perpetuate the negativism and close the doors to any further positive interaction. As an EMS manager, take the leadership role in attending medical society gatherings, and present the professional image of your organization as often as possible.

RELATIONS WITH HOSPITALS
AND NURSING HOMES

Another consumer group of special interest to an ambulance service falls into the patient-advocate category. Although not the actual user of the service, these people activate the EMS system on behalf of the patient. The manager needs to be sensitive to building relationships with this group.

The progressive manager will be aware of any potential conflicts before transporting patients to nursing homes and hospitals and develop procedures to expedite patient care for both. Radio communication of patient reports to receiving hospitals is not only for medical control, but also a courtesy announcement to the nursing staff. This simple courtesy allows a busy facility to better accommodate your client. The result? The patient is greeted like a guest and feels welcome. Another result is shorter service time for your unit. The EMS manager who encourages his staff to perform these courtesy communications to hospitals and nursing homes will spend less time defending his crew members' impatient toe-tapping behavior because they had to wait.

Encouraging your people to be friendly, personal and service-oriented toward hospitals and nursing home staffs will improve both working and human relations for your service, other agencies and most important for the patient.

The common educational interests of the hospital or nursing-home staff with your personnel may serve as a bridge builder. Planning for joint in-services, when appropriate, allows for these groups to share in a less stressful and neutral environment. Simply taking the unit to a nursing home to explain the services that your organization provides boosts staff morale, as well as informs and instructs participants from both organizations.

The Care and Feeding of Ambulance-Board Directors

Overview

The board of directors, or advisory board, of an EMS service can provide a unique contribution. The individual board members have different backgrounds and experiences to supply a fresh perspective to your management team. Of course, some boards are better informed and more enlightened than others. No matter what kind of board or advisory council your service is linked to, you need to make the best of it. This means *working* at developing a good relationship, providing a professional image and *always* being prepared.

In working with the board, always keep in mind that the perspective of the individual members will likely differ from yours. Learn to anticipate their reactions by trying to view how events and circumstances of the EMS service will affect them and their obligations and responsibilities to the community.

WHAT A BOARD UNIQUELY BRINGS

The board of directors contributes the following:

An objectivity that gives you a total overview of the organization with the ability to see the many parts as an integrated whole, not only as separate parts.

A freedom from the day-to-day operational pressures and concerns. This freedom enables focusing on creative visions for the future.

A firsthand awareness of the needs, concerns and interests of your customers and community. Knowledgeable board members are usually aware of the attitudes, rhythms, norms and value systems of their community.

A knowledge of the resources in the community.

A sense of history of the organization that provides consistency, stability and a sharp sense of mission and purpose.

An image of objectivity and trustworthiness the community gives the board. A board is entrusted to represent and act on its constituency's needs and desires. The public entrusts to the board its faith that it will be objective.

A questioning role that makes possible and mandatory the probing of the organization's assumptions and illusions. (For example, is success a beautiful new building or a reduction in response times to those served? What *is* success?)

A competent board is aware of what it brings to the organization and tends to exercise its power toward fulfilling its role. It hires a competent executive to manage the organization and then respects his or her ability to do so by not becoming involved in day-to-day operational issues.

DUTIES OF BOARD MEMBERS

The main responsibilities of an ambulance board of directors include the following:

1. Approving or initiating goals and major policies, long-range planning and strategies of the organization.
2. Assuring compliance with all legal requirements.

3. Assuring that sufficient capital is always available for effective operations.
4. Authorizing large expenditures, including contracts and other commitments, and maintaining physical assets.
5. Selecting and engaging the manager and approving promotions of key personnel.
6. Maintaining suitable organizational structure.
7. Providing leadership to the organization through the manager and through example.
8. Ensuring that the constituents they represent are dealt with fairly.
9. Evaluating achieved results, and maintaining control by asking the right questions and referring to regular reports from the manager.

TECHNIQUES FOR WORKING WITH BOARDS

There are many unemployed EMS managers who will attest to the importance of understanding how a relationship with a board must be developed and maintained.

Preparation is the single most important element of survival. A well-prepared manager is not surprised or ruffled by off-the-wall questions. Regular meeting times and places (for example, the first Tuesday of every month) are appreciated by busy board members who find it easier to attend if meetings are regularly scheduled. Material to be discussed should be well-prepared, brief and circulated in advance.

Chairpersons should be strong allies. They can be a manager's sounding board and shield him from "cheap shots" from other members. It's wise to meet with the chairperson at least two days in advance to confirm the actual agenda. Agenda order can have a significant effect on the outcome of a particular issue. In fact, it's wise to contact every board member before a meeting (possibly by phone) to make sure there are no surprises at the meeting.

Finally, minutes of the meeting should reflect what occurred, but need not be taken down word for word. It's more effective if the manager can write the board minutes to translate into action for recognition by the board.

Regulatory Agencies

Overview

There are a variety of regulatory agencies with which every EMS service must work. These organizations include EMS state offices or their equivalent, federal agencies like the Occupational Health and Safety Administration (OSHA), the U.S. Department of Labor's Wage and Hour Division, the Equal Employment Opportunity Commission (EEO), unemployment agencies, civil service commissions and local business licensing agencies, to name just a few. Federal, state or local legislation empowers these agencies to regulate. Most have wide powers that, when exercised, can bring any service to a standstill or tie up administrative personnel for months in hearings or fact-finding procedures.

It's important for a manager to know which agencies have jurisdiction or influence over the ambulance service's operations. After all, their purpose is to encourage or demand compliance with the laws themselves and the regulations used to interpret those laws. Should a question arise, a copy of all applicable regulations should be available at the ambulance service's headquarters for quick review by the manager. The manager must also decide what steps are necessary to comply with agency regulations.

GETTING ALONG WITH REGULATORS

They're not bad folks! Really! They are, however, committed to fair enforcement of applicable laws and regulations. The best way to get along is to comply—being on the wrong side of a powerful official is no fun. If your operation is in compliance, there's no reason to fear these officials.

Respect is another good word to remember when dealing with regulatory officials. Regulators don't appreciate being treated like lepers or as though they're coming to repossess your automobile. They expect EMS personnel to respect their position and the agency they represent. It never hurts to be gracious.

If there's a problem, be honest and demonstrate your personal commitment to an immediate resolution of the issue. The manager's credibility is extremely important here. If the regulator isn't strictly bound by his regulatory powers and at the same time can recognize a personal commitment by the manager, an agreeable resolution can follow.

A state-agency director relates this example:

> A manager called me last year to tell me that they were temporarily in violation of a minor regulation and what action was being taken to correct the problem. I was flabbergasted that they called to tell us they were in violation. In fact, our enforcement division was understaffed due to an illness, and would have never discovered the problem. That manager's honesty impressed me.

The next time that manager called to report a minor violation because of an equipment problem, the director loaned him the piece of equipment his service needed until he could get it fixed. The director said he realized they were working hard to comply with the regulations and said he thought it was appropriate to help. The moral: given a proper relationship, officials can be a source of information and a valuable resource for the EMS manager.

Developing
Team Support

Overview

Few health organizations have the pressure of providing service in such public places as restaurants, theaters, football stadiums and congested street intersections. But in EMS, these places and more, are the marketing arena! Your organization provides services in a highly visible environment, and is, therefore, assessed by numerous non-medical bystanders. What picture does your group paint? Is it compatible with the image you or your governing body expect? There are several ways to market your organization in the community. Most of these involve spending. Advertisements such as bumper stickers, billboards and newspaper ads are effective but can quickly drain your budget. In addition, all of these items will eventually fade from memory. It's important at this point to distinguish advertising from image. Advertising doesn't necessarily create a positive image or improve a poor one. On the contrary, advertising produces good results if a positive image has already been established.

The first step in assessing your image is to look around.

(continued on next page)

(continued)

The gleaming, freshly washed exterior of the ambulance is what will first catch your eye. After all, that's the only image of your organization many members of the community will ever have. Is there a clear, striking logo that's easy to remember? Was the vehicle driven courteously? Does your crew always appear well-groomed and neatly dressed in crisp uniforms? Murphy's law does prevail—it'll be the sloppy or incompetent person who'll enter the mayor's home on an emergency call. So be prepared.

If, as you look around, you aren't pleased with what you see, you can bet the public will feel the same way. Building a positive image starts internally. A manager must put his house in order before entering the public arena. Policy and procedure manuals will convey to team members the image they're expected to project, but management's consistent example and positive reinforcement will emphasize its importance and help to confirm it.

COMMUNITY INVOLVEMENT

Another excellent way to build a positive image with both your personnel and the public is for the organization to become an active participant in the community. Do members of management sit on boards of allied community organizations such as the Heart Association? Red Cross? Salvation Army? Are they involved with other community groups that could be strong supporters of EMS such as Rotary, Jaycees, Kiwanis or other service organizations? Does the service have representation in both political camps in the community? If management represents the service every time it attends or participates in these organizations' meetings, then the service becomes a true part of the community fabric. Its voice is then heard, respected and requested. It's also crucially important to develop a support network within the community to help with subsidies, to help during budget-cutting time or to help at any other time when you may need to gather financial or political support.

COMMUNITY EDUCATION

Developing a community-education or relations program will create a mechanism for public education, reflect an increase in company revenue and promote positive communication within the EMS system. Taking the lead in the community to educate all ages about the process of calling for an ambulance, and what to expect when the ambulance arrives, will generate awareness and interest about the service your company provides. Employee morale will also be boosted through participation in such programs.

Programs of this nature include junior paramedic programs, blood-pressure screening, sponsoring scouting groups and safety awards.

Options for these community programs are limited only by the team's creativity and imagination. Second only to providing patient care is building a positive image. It can be the most important external activity that you do.

MARKETING IS NOT A FOUR-LETTER WORD

Every EMS organization (public, private and volunteer) needs to market its services. The amount and *type* of marketing will depend on each organization's mission. EMS managers must be marketing oriented. The term marketing embraces selling and includes analysis, promotion and coordination.

The customer isn't necessarily the patient. For example, the city council or hospital can contract for services. Both customer and patient needs must be established by research. This research should be a continuous process and the manager should keep a detailed file of ideas, concepts and materials used by other services.

Promotion begins with internal items such as uniforms and organizational logos and may include sophisticated advertising created by public relations firms or consultants. There are numerous opportunities for free publicity. For example, one service had their name *tastefully* lettered on the back of each of the service's lightweight jackets in scotchlight letters. Each time the service's personnel were photographed at night while kneeling over a patient, the service's name was prominently featured on the front page of the newspaper.

In promoting your EMS organization throughout the community, consider these ideas, then add your own.

1. Issue your own small newsletter to customers. If it's well-done, you'll create reader interest and good will with chatty news while advertising your message. It will wind up in doctors' offices, banks, homes, and so on.

2. Speak at local club meetings. What's your message to the Rotary or Kiwanis? To the women's club? To a youth group?

3. Write press releases for local newspapers and radio on how many generations your family has been in the business, on your employees and on your services.

4. Publish instructive booklets connected with your services. Examples: "How to Handle an Emergency," "What Every Babysitter Should Know," "CPR," "First Aid Guide."

5. Encourage employees to promote your service among friends and relatives.

6. Create a local support group to tell what's good about your services. One service used an over-50 council to review services for seniors.

7. Arrange get-acquainted events. Invite the public to tour your headquarters. Give them small mementos of the visit.

8. Arrange educational displays about your service in your local library, banks, stockbrokers' offices and schools.

9. Merge your advertising with that of related but non-competitive organizations in cooperative mailings.

10. Sponsor athletic teams in your town. Every T-shirt or sweater emblazoned with your service's name on it is obviously great advertising but also illustrates you care about your community.

11. With each invoice include some piece of sales literature. You're paying the postage anyway, so put your latest message right in your customer's hands.

12. Provide community prizes for the high-school safe driver, for the scholarship winner, the most valuable player, the fishing-contest winner.

C A S E   S T U D Y   # 10

Medic Ambulance—A Community Celebration

Your ambulance company has had a membership program for the past three years. The first two years of the program showed a considerable increase in the number of new members, but last year's program showed a decline in renewals and only a marginal increase in new members.

Your review of the data indicates that although the number of new subscribers was increasing, the number of renewals had been decreasing over the three-year period. You realize that your board of directors is unhappy with the program's performance, and you've taken the problem to your staff for input and suggestions. They developed a strategy that will address the issue. You will present their program, "Medic Ambulance—A Community Celebration," to the board for their endorsement and participation, in what will be a gala event.

Goal:

A celebration to kick off the first day of the 1987 membership drive, that focuses the community and media on Medic Ambulance Service.

Objectives:

1. To increase community visibility of Medic Ambulance Service.
2. To obtain 80 percent renewal memberships from last year.
3. To generate a 20 percent increase in new memberships.
4. To provide the community with information regarding emergency care.
5. To demonstrate Medic Ambulance's lead role in coordinating health-care resources in the community.

You've budgeted $4,000 for the event, which will be offset by the projected $7,000 in direct-membership revenues, $5,500 in projected new-members' use of the ambulance service in the upcoming year that is expected to result from the event. There will also be an indirect revenue effect from the marketing and the visibility of the ambulance service in the community, although this impact is not easily measured.

Preliminary discussions initiated by you and your staff with local hospitals, nursing homes, and health groups demonstrate their interest in having one community education day that would focus on health care. Your service's experience and willingness to coordinate the event has heightened the interest of these groups to participate, should a community celebration be held.

Your staff has suggested that the program would have the greatest attendance on a Sunday afternoon, immediately following church hours. A time period from 1:00 p.m. to 6:00 p.m. would allow for the most efficient use of time for maximum exposure to the public and media. The date selected is June 4, as it's the first Sunday following Memorial Day, and historically a slow day for the media.

The program is designed as a health-fair setting, with brief sessions directed at providing public education. Programs sponsored by Medic Ambulance Service will include baby-sitter training, demonstration of the Heimlich maneuver, Junior Paramedic classes, the Trauma Teddy program, and blood-pressure screening. Local hospitals and health groups will be participating with booths that will highlight the services that they provide to the community.

The program highlights, as outlined to the board, include the following:

1. A kickoff and toast to community members who have supported Medic Ambulance throughout the years.
2. Special recognition to the staffs of each of the community's hospitals and nursing homes.
3. Testimonials from Medic Ambulance staff members about public-safety services, citing incidents where support from police, fire and sheriff departments have been outstanding.
4. Testimonials from current members regarding the service they received from Medic Ambulance.
5. Recognition of local journalists who have provided the community with objective reporting. This is further supported by a display of news articles in a collage or video-tape recordings of broadcasts.
6. Special recognitions and announcements from ambulance board members will be held throughout the course of the day for staff members of Medic Ambulance.
7. Tours of the ambulances and the communications center.
8. Tours of the computer and billing offices where members can watch their names being entered onto the computer.
9. An area will be set aside to view the Medic Ambulance slide presentation.

Refreshments will be served, including punch and a large sheet cake bearing the Medic Ambulance logo and the outline of communities served, with each of the health centers, hospitals and nursing homes listed on the cake.

The program will feature prominent government figures from the community, and members of the community at large, both of which tend to draw media attention.

■ ■ ■

THE DIFFERENCE BETWEEN
MARKETING AND ADVERTISING

Marketing implies total promotion of the service, including community education and involvement. *Advertising* uses specific items that help influence the customer to use a particular service. Traditionally, these have included phone stickers, letters, brochures, telephone-message pads, pens or pencils, calendars, and so on. Newspaper advertising, electronic advertising and billboards are occasionally used by services in larger communities.

Many political subdivisions are beginning to look at marketing their services the same way private ambulance services have done for years. They're desperate to develop other mechanisms to support emergency services. Some of these have included positioning the public service to also handle non-emergency transfers with excess production capacity, developing new service lines such as fixed-wing service or wheel-chair service and, finally, providing training (for profit) for other agencies.

There is no bigger hero in government than an EMS manager who can tell the city council, "We've lowered response times, increased the quality of care, and need 50 percent less subsidy this year." Council members will sit up and take notice!!

And Finally. . . The Never-ending Journey

Emergency medical service is changing. Be ready for the changes and challenges ahead. We believe that the best way to predict the future, as an EMS leader, is to create it. Today, with requests for service increasing, and dollars available to perform the service decreasing, managers have to be constantly alert in their search for a "better EMS mousetrap."

Public and private services alike are discovering incredible untapped resources right in their own backyards—their employees. What does it take to develop this resource? It takes managers and leaders willing to create the future of EMS by knowing how to organize, inspire, and empower others to achieve their organization's goals.

There's nothing revolutionary in the fundamentals being taught about effective management and leadership. People have been inspiring other people (leadership) and creating systems for performance evaluation (management) since the first hunters realized a little teamwork could pull down a woolly mammoth.

What *is* revolutionary is the new-found interest in *applying* these principles. The companies that compete successfully today have taken these fundamental lessons to heart and practice them faithfully. Other organizations, whether non-profit government or private enterprise, have begun to realize that if they want more productivity from fewer people, they have to make these people *want* to work to their fullest potential. And they do this by creating an environment where people feel a part of the team and believe that what they're doing is making a difference.

There are lots of special skills people need to acquire in order to become effective leaders and managers. They can *all* be taught to some degree. Working their way up through management, many of today's leaders wished they'd known more about some of these skills. After reading this far, you're obviously one of those interested in learning new skills, or perhaps improving existing skills, in order to go "beyond the street,"—interested in becoming the best leader you can be. Among the many skills discussed throughout this book, five stand out. The following five skills summarize what we feel will help you realize that best part of yourself to become the best leader you can be.

People Skills. First, if you like working alone, and you're not too fond of Homo sapiens, do everyone a favor and *don't* become a manager. You have to sincerely like people if you're going to be effective at organizing and motivating them. People skills are the most important tools a supervisor can bring to the job. It's what makes people work harder and feel good about it. They can tell by your actions that you care about their well-being and that you respect their role in helping the organization reach its goals. Outstanding managers show that they care about their people's continued professional development and are sensitive to their special needs. They learn to be patient and to value what people being to their jobs, beyond technical skills.

Administrative Skills. Do you find yourself taking on duties or projects because "If I want it done right, I'd better do it myself"? If so, you need help! As a manager, you *have* to depend on others, whether or not they can do something as well as you. The art of delegating includes knowing when its appropriate and then providing the proper guidelines and authority to accomplish the task. An old Japanese proverb says that if you give someone a fish, he'll eat *today.* If you teach him how to fish, he'll eat for a *lifetime.* You'll be doing both yourself and your colleagues a favor if you properly delegate.

Communications Skills. Are you a good listener? On the street, you can't always focus your attention on the person talking to you. When minutes are critical, a dozen different considerations will compete for your attention. When not in the field, however, you don't have that excuse. Learn to be a good listener, and force yourself to stop and focus on what's being said. If someone is long-winded and taking up valuable time, don't start on paperwork and say, "Go ahead, I'm listening." You're not, and they know it. You're better off concentrating on how to get them to come to the point. Sometimes simply standing up is an effective way to signal that you need to go and are concluding the conversation.

Public speaking and writing skills are a critical part of communicating well. And both can be mastered, or at least learned, with practice, practice, practice. If you're presently not doing much of either, take the time to do so. Speaking in front of people is nerve-racking at first, and writing, like thinking, is hard, but doing both well will give you a significant edge.

Political Savvy. There are no formal classes in political skills, but if you don't develop this sixth sense now, you'll never survive as a leader. Critical to this skill is an acute sense of timing—knowing where and when to fight, as well as when not to.

Do you hate politics and bureaucracies? Most of us do, but they're a fact of life. You don't have to like them, but you do have to know the rules if you're going to be effective. There's a network within every geopolitical group, and the successful manager knows when and how to access it. One more hint. In our collective experience, we've found that the bureaucrats consider *timeliness* next to godliness. If you agree to complete a project by a certain time, do it!

Personal Attributes. You might be surprised to discover that your employees will forgive you a variety of sins in management technique if they believe in *you.* Your basic integrity, honesty and warmth will come through loud and clear, overshadowing any mismanagement or human error.

•   •   •

When these five skills are learned and used in an EMS organization, the results can be amazing. People discover an excitement in the mission of the organization. They gain a wider view of their organization and the importance of their individual contributions. Through increased involvement, people are enthused toward greater creativity, capability and productivity.

There's no perfect candidate for an EMS leader. Effective supervisors and leaders understand both their strengths and weaknesses, and compensate for those they don't do well. The development of management and leadership skills is a never-ending journey—but there is no reward greater than knowing your leadership skills have helped others reach their potential, and your organization reach its goals. Life "beyond the street" isn't easy, but it's worth it!

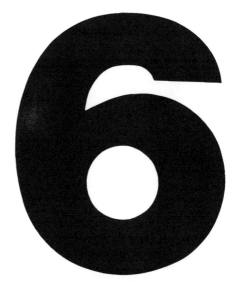

P A R T

Appendices

A P P E N D I X   A

EMS Locker-Room Lingo

A Glossary of Ambulance Operations, Communications, Legal and Reimbursement Terminology

— A —

ACCEPT ASSIGNMENT: Providers of medical care may choose to directly bill a third-party payer and receive payment directly from the third party. Under Medicare, the beneficiary need not pay any difference between actual charges and those charges deemed reasonable by Medicare when the provider accepts assignment. However, the beneficiary must still pay any deductible and co-insurance.

ACTUAL CHARGE: A charge made by an ambulance service for a specific service at a specific time. The actual charge may not reflect the customary charge.

ACUTE CARE: Care for victims of acute disease or injury or acute exacerbation of chronic disease. Acute care provision requires availability of a comprehensive array of services and skills and concentrated continuous care.

ACUTE DISEASE: A disease which is characterized by a single episode of fairly short duration from which the patient returns to his normal or previous state and level of activity.

ADMINISTRATIVE AGENCY: An arm of government which administers or carries out legislation. For example, Workmen's Compensation Commission.

ADMISSIBILITY (of evidence): Evidence that meets the legal rules of evidence and can go to the jury.

ADVANCED LIFE SUPPORT (ALS): For ambulance services, includes the services of basic life support (BLS) and advanced emergency care. Ambulance personnel use these services: intravenous therapy, esophageal obturator, endotracheal airway, anti-shock trousers, cardiac monitor (EKG), cardiac defibrillator, drugs, relief of pneumothorax or other advanced procedures and services.

AFFIDAVIT: A voluntary sworn statement of facts, or a voluntary declaration in writing of fact, that a person swears to be true before an official authorized to administer an oath.

AGENCY: The relationship in which one person acts for or represents another. For example, employer and employee.

ALL-INCLUSIVE RATE: A flat fee charged for services rendered.

ALLEGATION: A statement that a person expects to prove.

ALLOWABLE CHARGE: Generic term referring to the maximum fee that a third party will use in reimbursing a provider for a given service.

ALLOWABLE COSTS: Items or elements of a provider's costs which are reimbursable under a payment formula. Medicare, Medicaid and most Blue Cross plans reimburse services for certain costs, but do not allow reimbursement for all costs.

ALS: Advanced life support.

ANTENNA: A system of wires or electrical conductors for reception or transmission of radio waves. Specifically, a radiator which couples the transmission line or lead-in to space, for transmission or reception of electromagnetic radio waves. (Also known as aerial.)

ASSIGNMENT OF BENEFITS: Written authorization by a subscriber permitting payment of benefits directly to a provider. (See ACCEPT ASSIGNMENT.)

AUDIO: Frequencies corresponding to a normally audible sound wave. The voice component of the transmitted signal. The normal ear responds to audio frequencies.

— B —

BAD DEBTS: Amounts considered to be uncollectable from accounts and notes receivable which were created or acquired in providing services.

BASE STATION: An item of fixed radio hardware consisting of a transmitter and a receiver. A land station in the land-mobile service carrying on a service with land-mobile stations.

BASIC LIFE SUPPORT (BLS): For ambulance service, includes only transportation, first aid and any needed administration of oxygen.

BATTERY: The touching of one person by another without permission.

BEST-EVIDENCE RULE: A legal doctrine requiring that primary evidence of a fact (such as an original document) be introduced, or at least explained, before a copy can be introduced or testimony given concerning the fact.

BLS: Basic life support.

BLUE CROSS (BC): A nonprofit, tax-exempt health service prepayment organization providing coverage for health-care (hospital) and related services.

BLUE SHIELD (BS): A nonprofit, tax-exempt medical service prepayment organization providing for medical care (physician) and related services.

BONA FIDE: In good faith; openly, honestly or innocently; without knowledge or intent of fraud.

BORROWED SERVANT: An employee temporarily under the control of another. The traditional example is that of a nurse employed by a hospital who is borrowed by a surgeon in the operating room. The temporary employer of the borrowed servant will be held responsible for the act of the borrowed servant under the doctrine of respondent superior.

— C —

CARRIER (communications): Radio wave radiated by a transmitter without modulation.

CARRIER (reimbursement): A commercial insurance firm or Blue Shield plan administering Part B of Medicare. It is distinguished from commercial insurance companies or Blue Cross plans administering Part A, which are referred to as intermediaries.

CASH DISCOUNT: Reduction in cash payment granted for settlement of debt within a stipulated period.

CHANNEL: Sometimes used synonymously with frequency. It is the electronic signal path through which radio frequencies flow.

CHANNEL RADIO: An assigned band of frequencies of sufficient width to permit its use for radio communication. The necessary width of a channel depends on the type of transmission and the tolerance for the frequency of emission.

CIVIL LAW: The law of countries such as Germany and France which follow the Roman law system of jurisprudence in which law is enacted. It is also the portion of American law which does not deal with crimes.

CLAIM: A request to an insurer by an insured person or his assignee for payment of benefits under an insurance policy.

CLOSED-SHOP CONTRACT: A labor-management agreement which provides that only members of a particular union may be hired.

CO-CHANNEL INTERFERENCE: Interference caused by other parties using the same transmitting frequency already being used.

CO-INSURANCE: Established percentages indicating the portion of covered expenses, beyond the deductible, to be paid under the coverage and the portion to be borne by the subscriber (patient).

COMMERCIALS: Usually used to refer to all private insurers except Blue Cross and Blue Shield.

COMMON LAW: The legal traditions of England and the United States where part of the law is developed by court decisions.

COMMUNICATIONS LINK: Established communications between two parties. Example: emergency program manager to units on scene.

COMMUNICATIONS NETWORK: A combination of links that are complete as to some specific function. Examples: A network to serve command personnel. A network to serve air-to-air control.

CONFIDENTIAL INFORMATION: See PRIVILEGED COMMUNICATION.

CONSENT: A voluntary act by which one person agrees to allow someone else to do something. For medical liability purposes, consents should be in writing with an explanation of the procedures to be performed.

CONTINUOUS DUTY: A rating applied to receivers and transmitters to indicate their capability for use in a continuous-duty cycle (as opposed to the term intermittent duty).

CONTRACTUAL ALLOWANCE: An accounting adjustment to reflect the difference between charges for services rendered to insured persons and the amount paid for those services under contract with the third-party payer.

CONTROL CONSOLE: A desk-mounted enclosed panel which contains a number of controls used to operate a radio station.

CO-PAYMENT: A type of health care cost-sharing whereby the insured or covered person pays a fixed amount per unit of medical service or unit of time (for example, $2 per physician visit, $10 per inpatient hospital day) and the insurer pays the rest of the cost. The co-payment is incurred at the time the service is used, and the amount paid does not vary with the cost of the service (unlike co-insurance, which is payment of some percentage of the cost).

COUNTERCLAIM: A defendant's claim against the plaintiff.

COVERAGE: In a radio communications system, the geographic area where reliable communications exist; usually expressed in terms of miles extending radially from a fixed radio station.

CRIMINAL LAW: The division of the law dealing with crime and punishment.

CUSTOMARY CHARGE: Used interchangeably with the term usual charge and referring to that amount the provider normally and usually charges the majority of patients for a particular medical service.

— D —

DECEDENT: A dead person.

DECIBEL (db): A unit which expresses the level of a power value relative to a reference power value. Specifically, the level of a power value P relative to a reference value PR in decibels is defined as $10 \log 10$ (p/Pr).

DEFAMATION: The injury of a person's reputation or character by willful and malicious statements made to a third person. Defamation includes libel and slander.

DEFENDANT: In a criminal case, the person accused of committing a crime. In a civil suit, the party against whom suit is brought demanding that he pay the other party legal relief.

DEPOSITION: A sworn statement, made out of court, which may be admitted into evidence if it is impossible for a witness to attend in person.

DIAGNOSIS-RELATED GROUP (DRG): Classification procedure adapted from a Yale University study representing 467 major diagnostic categories (MDC) which aggregates patients into case types based upon diagnosis. A diagnosis-related group is a subset of a major diagnostic category. Under the prospective-payment system, Medicare uses the 467 DRGs for basis of payment.

DIRECT COST: A cost which is identifiable directly with a particular activity, service or product.

DIRECTED VERDICT: When a trial judge decides that the evidence or law is so clearly in favor of one party that it is pointless for the trial to proceed further. The judge directs the jury to return a verdict for that party.

DISCOVERY: Pretrial activities when attorneys determine what evidence the opposing side will present if the case comes to trial. Discovery prevents attorneys from being surprised during trial and facilitates out-of-court settlement.

DRG: See DIAGNOSIS-RELATED GROUP.

DUMPING: Interhospital transfer of uninsured, poorly insured (Medicaid) or complicated patients, for reasons which are primarily financial and not related to the need for medical services available only at the receiving institution.

DUPLEX OPERATION: The simultaneous transmitting and receiving of apparatus at one location in conjunction with associated transmitting and receiving equipment at another location. The operation of associated transmitting and receiving apparatus concurrently as in ordinary telephones without manual switching between talking and listening periods. A separate frequency band is required for each direction of transmission.

DUPLEXER: A device which is used in radio equipment to provide simultaneous transmit and receive (full-duplex operation) on a single antenna.

— E —

ECF: Extended-care facility.

EKG: Electrocardiogram. A visual representation of heart muscle electrical activity.

EMERGENCY CALLS: Refers to all calls in which an ambulance is dispatched to an unschduled destination for a possible emergency. Related terms include the following:
    Non-Emergency Calls: Refers to all scheduled transfers.
    Response: Request for service where unit is dispatched.
    Transport: Incident in which actual patient trasportation occurs.

EMT: Emergency medical technician. A person licensed to perform basic life-support and first-aid procedures.

EMT-P: See PARAMEDIC.

EXPERT WITNESS: One who has special training, experience, skill and knowledge in a relevant area and who is allowed to offer an opinion as testimony in court.

EXTENDED-CARE FACILITY: Organizations with medical staffs and continuous professional nursing services that provide comprehensive short-term inpatient care (usually post-acute hospital care). They also serve convalescent patients who are not acutely ill, or who are in a stable state of illness with a variety of medical conditions.

— F —

FEE-FOR-SERVICE: A method of reimbursing for services rendered. In an insurance plan, such as Blue Shield, a schedule of benefits covered is prepared and a fee is established for each benefit. This becomes the fee-for-service. This definition can also be applied to non-insured patients (self-pay) or benefits not covered by insurance plans. In this case, a schedule of services and fees would be available at the location rendering the service. This is the usual method of billing by the majority of the country's ambulance services.

FREE-STANDING FACILITY: An ambulatory care facility that has no physical connection with a hospital or other health-care unit. Normally, a free-standing facility is far from other health-care facilities.

FREQUENCY: The number of complete cycles per unit of time. When the unit of time is one second, the measurement unit is hertz (cycles per second).

FREQUENCY BAND: A continuous range of frequencies extending between two limiting frequencies.

FREQUENCY MODULATION (FM): A method of modulating a carrier-frequency signal by causing the frequency accordance with the intelligence signal to be transmitted. The amount of deviation in frequency above and below the resting frequency is at each intelligence signal being transmitted. The number of complete deviations per second above and below the resting frequency corresponds at each instant to the frequency of the intelligence signal being transmitted.

— G —

GEOGRAPHIC ASSIGNMENT: The assignment and use of communications channels on a dedicated-user basis within a given geographic area.

GOOD-SAMARITAN LAW: A legal doctrine designed to protect those who stop voluntarily to render aid in an emergency.

— H —

HALF-DUPLEX CHANNEL: A communications channel providing duplex operation at one end of the channel but not at the other. Typically, the base station is operated in the duplex mode. (For comparison, see SIMPLEX CHANNEL.)

HEALTH CARE FINANCING ADMINISTRATION (HCFA): A principal operating component of the Department of Health and Human Services composed of organizational units with responsibilities related to the administration of Medicare, Medicaid and their supporting functions and services.

HEALTH MAINTENANCE ORGANIZATION (HMO): Any organization that, through an organized system of health care, provides or assures the delivery of an agreed set of comprehensive health maintenance and treatment services for an enrolled group of persons under a prepaid fixed sum or payment-per-capita arrangement. Services available usually include primary care and rehabilitation. HMOs are also known as prepaid health plans. The HMO must employ or contract with health-care providers who undertake a continuing responsibility to provide services to its enrollees. To be considered a federally qualified Health Maintenance Organization, the HMO must meet the provisions of Title XIII of the Public Health Service Act.

HIGH-BAND VHF: Radio frequencies from 142 to 174 MHz

— I —

IN LOCO PARENTIS: A legal doctrine under which certain circumstances the courts may assign a person to stand in place of parents and possess their legal rights, duties, and responsibilities toward a child.

INDEPENDENT CONTRACTOR: One who agrees to undertake work without being under the direct control or direction of the employer.

INDICTMENT: A formal written criminal accusation brought by a prosecuting attorney against one charged with criminal conduct.

INDIRECT COST: A cost which cannot be identified directly with a particular activity, service, or product of the program experiencing the cost. Indirect costs are usually apportioned among the program's services in proportion to each service's share of direct costs.

INJUNCTION: A court order requiring a person to do or not to do a certain act.

INTERFERENCE: Interference in a signal transmission path is either extraneous power (which results in loss of signal) or distortion of information.

INTERMEDIARY: An organization selected by health-care providers which has entered in an agreement with the Department of Health and Human Services under Medicare's hospital insurance program (Part A) to process claims and perform other functions. Usually, but not necessarily, a Blue Cross plan or private insurance company, it is distinguished from commercial insurance companies or Blue Shield plans administering Part B, which are referred to as carriers.

INTERMEDIATE-CARE FACILITY (ICF): An institution licensed under state law to provide, on a regular basis, health care and services to individuals who do not require the degree of care and treatment which a hospital or a skilled nursing facility is designed to provide. The individuals must, however, require care and services above the level of room and board. Federal payment for intermediate care-facility services is limited to Medicaid.

INTERROGATORIES: A list of questions sent from one party in a lawsuit to the other party to be answered.

— L —

LAND MOBILE: Communications between base stations and mobile radios or from mobile radio to mobile radio.

LIABILITY: An obligation one has incurred or might incur through any act or failure to act.

LIABILITY INSURANCE: A contract to have someone else pay for any liability or loss in return for the payment of premiums.

LIBEL: A published or broadcast communication that lowers a person's reputation through scorn, ridicule or contempt.

LICENSE: A permit from the state allowing certain acts to be performed, usually for a specific period of time.

LITIGATION: A trial in court to determine legal issues, rights and duties between the parties involved.

LONG-TERM CARE (LTC): Includes all forms of services, both institutional and non-institutional, that are required by people with chronic health conditions. Such conditions may be experienced at any age as recurrent or persistent symptoms, illness, disability or impairment of a physical or mental nature.

LOW-BAND VHF: Radio frequencies from 30 to 50 MHz.

— M —

MALPRACTICE: Professional misconduct, improper discharge of professional duties or failure to meet the standard of care of a professional which results in harm to another.

MEDICAID: As authorized by Title XIX of the Social Security Act, Medicaid is a federally assisted program, operated and administered by individual states, which provides medical benefits for eligible low-income people (those who are members of one of the categories of people who can be covered under welfare case-payment programs), the aged, blind, disabled and members of families with dependent children, where one parent is absent, incapacitated or unemployed. Under certain circumstances, states may provide Medicaid coverage for children under 21 who are not categorically related. Subject to broad federal guidelines, states define covered benefits, eligibility, rates of payment to providers and methods of program administration.

MEDICAL CONTROL TERMINAL: A unit of electronic equipment located in hospital emergency rooms or cardiac-care units which displays EKGs and records voices and data received from an EMS scene by transmission via radio or telephone.

MEDICAL DIRECTOR: The physician under whose license and authority EMTs and paramedics provide services.

MEDICAL CONTROL: The hospital designated to give radio instructions to ambulance crews.

MEDICARE: Title XVIII of the Social Security Act of 1965, which assists in payment for medical and health services for persons age 65 and over, for persons eligible for Social Security disability payments for over two years. Health insurance protection is available to insured persons without regard to income. The major benefits of this legislation include physician services, hospital care, home care, and extended-care-facility coverage for a defined period of time. This program is financed through Social Security deductions from employee-employer payrolls and is handled through national trust funds. Part A covers hospital and skilled nursing-facility costs. Part B, for which there is a monthly premium, covers physician services and is processed through insurance companies that serve as intermediaries and carriers.

MEGAHERTZ (MHz): A common technical term that refers to the frequency of the radio—1 MHz = 1,000,000 cycles per second or hertz.

MICROWAVE: Radio waves in the frequency range of 1,000 MHz and upward. Generally defines operations in the region where boundaries are used instead of conventional lumped-constant circuit components.

MISDEMEANOR: An unlawful act of a less serious nature than a felony, usually punishable by fine or imprisonment for a term of less than one year.

MOBILE RELAY STATION: A fixed station established for the automatic retransmission of mobile service radio communications which originate on the transmitting frequency of the mobile stations and which are retransmitted on the receiving frequency of the mobile stations.

MOBILE UNIT: A two-way radio-equipped vehicle or person. Also, sometimes the two-way radio itself, when associated with a vehicle or person.

MODULATION: The process of modifying some characteristic of an electromagnetic wave (called a carrier) so that it varies in step with instantaneous value of another wave (called a modulating wave or signal). The carrier can be a direct current, an alternating current (providing its frequency is above the highest frequency component in the modulating wave), or a series of regular repeating, uniform pulses called a pulse chain (providing their repetition rate is at least twice that of the highest frequency to be transmitted).

MONITOR: To listen to mobile radio messages without transmitting.

MULTIPLEX OPERATION: Simultaneous transmission of two or more messages in either or both directions or the same transmission path.

— N —

NEGLIGENCE: Carelessness, failure to act as an ordinary prudent person, or action contrary to what a reasonable person would have done.

NON-ALLOWABLE CHARGE: A charge for services that is not recognized as payable by a third-party payer because the service is not covered under the plan. Also, charges for covered services which are above those allowed under reasonable, customary or prevailing charges.

— O —

OMNI-DIRECTIONAL ANTENNA: An antenna that radiates signals with equal strength in all directions.

ORDINANCE: A law passed by a municipal legislative body.

OUTPATIENT HOSPITAL SERVICES: Diagnostic, curative, rehabilitative or educational health care provided on a scheduled basis to patients who are not expected to be lodged in the hospital at midnight.

OUTPUT: The energy resulting from the work the radio performs. Power output: the strength of the signal as it leaves the transmitter. Audio output: the strength of the voice wave as it leaves the speaker. Both are usually measured in watts.

— P —

PARAMEDIC: An individual trained and licensed to perform advanced life-support procedures under the direction of a physician.

PATIENT MIX: The numbers and types of patients served by a hospital or other health program. Patients may be classified according to their geographic location, socioeconomic characteristics, diagnoses or severity of illness.

PERJURY: The willful act of giving false testimony under oath.

POINT-TO-POINT RADIO COMMUNICATIONS: Radio communication between two fixed stations.

POLICE POWER: The power of the state to protect health, safety, morals and general welfare.

PORTABLE/PERSONAL COMMUNICATIONS EQUIPMENT: Radio transmitters, receivers, or combinations of both, which can be hand carried or worn on the person and which are operated from their own portable power sources and antenna.

PORTABLE RADIO: A completely self-contained radio which may be moved from one place to another.

PREFERRED-PROVIDER ORGANIZATION (PPO): An insurance arrangement whereby insurers contract with providers for certain services based on a fee schedule. Plan members are then encouraged to use these preferred providers for necessary services. If the insured chooses to use the services of a provider other than one within the organization, the insured must himself pay (out-of-pocket) any difference between charges and the approved-fee schedule.

PREVAILING CHARGE: A charge which falls within the range of charges most frequently used in a locality for a particular medical service procedure. The upper limit of this range establishes an overall limitation on the charges which a Medicare carrier that considers prevailing charges in reimbursement will accept as reasonable for a given service, without adequate special justification.

PRIOR AUTHORIZATION: Requirement imposed by a third party, under some review system, that a provider must justify before a peer review committee, insurance company representative or state agent the need for delivering a particular service to a patient, before actually providing the service, in order to receive reimbursement. (Synonymous with preauthorization, precertification, predetermination.)

PRIVILEGED COMMUNICATION: Statement made to an attorney, physician, spouse or anyone else in a position of trust. Because of the confidential nature of such information, the law protects it from being revealed even in court. The term is applied in two distinct situations. First, the communications between certain persons, such as physicians and patient, cannot by divulged without consent of the patient. Second, in some situations the law provides an exemption from liability for disclosing information where there is a higher duty to speak, such as statutory reporting requirements.

PROBATE: The judicial proceeding which determines the existence and validity of a will.

PROBATE COURT: Court with jurisdiction over wills. Its powers range from deciding the validity of a will to distributing property.

PROSPECTIVE REIMBURSEMENT: Any method of paying hospitals or ambulance services in which amounts or rates of payment are established in advance for the coming year. The programs paid these amounts regardless of the costs actually incurred. These systems of reimbursement are designed to introduce a degree of constraint on charge or cost increase by setting limits on amount paid during a future period. (Synonymous with prospective payment.)

PROXIMATE: In immediate relation with something else. In negligence cases, the careless act must be a proximate cause of injury.

PUSH-TO-TALK OPERATION (PTT) (PRESS-TO-TALK): Communication over a speech circuit in which transmission occurs from only one station at a time, the talker being required to keep a switch operated while talking.

— R —

RADIO INTERFERENCE: Undesired disturbance of radio reception. Man-made interference is generated by electric devices, with the resulting interference signals either radiated through space as electromagnetic waves or traveling over power lines or other conducting media. Radiated inteference is also due to natural sources such as atmospheric phenomena (lightning). Radio transmitters themselves may interfere with each other.

RADIO-RELAY SYSTEM (RADIO RELAY): A point-to-point radio transmission system in which signals are received and retransmitted by one or more intermediate radio stations.

REAL-TIME ALLOCATIONS: The assignment and use of communications channels on an incident-by-incident basis.

REASONABLE CHARGE: Under Medicare, the lower of either the customary charge by a particular ambulance service for a particular medical service or the prevailing charge for the service in that geographical area. Reimbursement is based on the lower of the reasonable and actual charges.

RELAY STATION: Radio stations that rebroadcast signals the instant they are received, so that the signal can be passed onto another station outside the range of the originating transmitter.

REMOTE: A control, usually desk mounted, for operating a distantly located station transmitter.

REMOTE-CONTROL EQUIPMENT: The apparatus used for one-way or two-way communications signals and delivering corresponding signals which are either amplified or reshaped or both.

REPEATER CHANNEL: A two-frequency channel that uses an intermediate repeater to extend the range of the channel. The repeater unit simultaneously receives on one frequency and transmits on another. It is inefficient in that two distinct frequencies are required to establish one communications channel.

REPEATER STATION: An operational fixed station established for the automatic retransmission of radio communications received from any station in the mobile service.

— S —

SERS (SPECIAL EMERGENCY RADIO SERVICE): That portion of radio communications frequency resources authorized for use in the alleviation of emergency situations endangering life or property.

SKILLED-NURSING FACILITY (SNF): Under Medicare and Medicaid, an institution (or a distinct part of an institution) which has in effect a transfer agreement with one or more participating hospitals and is primarily engaged in providing skilled nursing care or rehabilitation services for patients who require medical or nursing care or rehabilitation. In an SNF, the health care of each patient must be supervised by a physician.

SIMPLEX CHANNEL: A communications channel providing transmission in one direction only at any given time.

SIMPLEX CHANNEL, SIGNAL FREQUENCY: A simplex channel using only one assigned band of frequencies. (For comparison see SIMPLEX CHANNEL, TWO-FREQUENCY.)

SIMPLEX CHANNEL, TWO-FREQUENCY: A simplex radio system using two distinct assigned bands of frequency. (For comparison see SIMPLEX CHANNEL, SIGNAL FREQUENCY.)

SIMPLEX OPERATION: A method of operation in which communication between two stations takes place in one direction at a time.

SINGLE-FREQUENCY CHANNEL: A channel which is direct from transmitter to receiver. Transmitter and receiver frequencies are identical.

SQUELCH: A circuit function that acts to suppress the audio output of a receiver when noise power that exceeds a predetermined level is present.

SQUELCH CONTROL: The control to eliminate receiver noise when no signal is being received. It should be set up to just eliminate this noise. Turning it further will reduce the receiving range of the receiver.

SUBCARRIER: A carrier used to generate a modulated wave which is applied, in turn, as a modulating wave to modulate another carrier.

SYSTEM-STATUS MANAGEMENT: A system to optimize deployment and use of ambulances. It is a computer system designed to assure appropriate response time and vehicle location to meet service demands with less resources.

— T —

TALK BACK: The transmission of radio communications from portable and mobile radios to a base radio.

TALK OUT: The transmission of radio communications from a base-station radio to mobile and portable radios.

TAX EQUITY AND FISCAL RESPONSIBILITY ACT (TEFRA): Federal legislation enacted in 1982 which relates to tax increases and tax reform and contains numerous provisions that affect Medicare and Medicaid. The health-related sections of the act provide for extensive changes in Medicare including the introduction of cost-per-case limits on inpatient cost reimbursement.

TELECOMMUNICATION: Communication at a distance, as in telegraph, telephone cable or electromagnetic radiation.

TELEPHONE PATCH: An instrument that allows a radio to be used as an entrance and exit point from the commercial telephone system.

TERTIARY CARE: Subspecialty care usually requiring facilities of university-affiliated or teaching hospitals that have extensive diagnostic and treatment capabilities.

THIRD-PARTY PAYER: Any organization, public or private, which pays or insures health or medical expenses on behalf of beneficiaries or recipients (for example, Blue Cross and Blue Shield, commercial insurance companies, Medicare and Medicaid). The individual generally pays a premium for such coverage in all private and some public programs. The organization then pays bills on the patient's behalf. Such payments are called third-party payments and are distinguished by the separations among the individual receiving the service (the first party), the individual or institution providing it (the second party), and the organization paying for it (the third party).

TONE: Tone as applied to a selective-signaling system is an audio or carrier of controlled amplitude and frequency.

TONE CODE: Tone code specifies the character of the transmitted tone signal required to effect a particular selection.

TRANSCEIVER: The combination of radio transmitting and receiving equipment in a common housing, usually for portable or mobile use, and employing common circuit components for both transmitting and receiving. Generally used in push-to-talk operation.

TRANSMISSION LINE: A material structure forming a continuous path from one place to another, for directing the transmission of electromagnetic energy along this path.

TWO-WAY RADIO: A radio which is able to both transmit and receive.

— U —

ULTRA-HIGH FREQUENCY (UHF): Radio frequency from 300 to 3000 MHz, the upper portion from about 1000 to 3000 MHz is often referred to as low-capacity microwave.

UNIT HOUR: Term used to describe one staffed ambulance hour. (This represents two man-hours.)

UNIT IDENTIFIER: An identifier is assigned by the licensee to a mobile station for exact identification as "Car 3" or "797," etc. Does not eliminate the need for FCC-assigned station identifier or call sign.

USUAL, CUSTOMARY AND REASONABLE (UCR): A method of payment which allows the ambulance service's usual charge as long as it does not exceed the customary allowance, or the amount customarily charged for the service by other ambulance services in the area, unless it is determined to be a reasonable amount for the services rendered.

— V —

VEHICULAR REPEATER: A vehicular unit that is used to relay signals to and from a radio remote to the vehicle.

— W —

WHIP: Term applied to the long, slender mobile antenna usually found mounted on the vehicle bumper.

Note: Terry L. Schmidt, Frank Foster, JD, and Mike Grey contributed to the definitions in this section. Their contributions are gratefully acknowledged.

A   P   P   E   N   D   I   X   B

Sample Disaster Plan — An Overview

The paramedic and emergency medical technician role at multi-casualty disasters becomes more of an organizational than a medical function. The role has evolved from a number of medical and legal sources with an emphasis on common sense and the need for flexibility.

A high priority must be to restore order to an often chaotic situation. This can be best accomplished through the implementation of a preplanned scenario by those first on the scene. Specific logistical roles are assigned to provide for the orderly and rapid transport of victims to medical facilities. Casualties must be quickly evacuated to hospitals and casualty collection points, must be established where adequate medical supplies and personnel are available. Only in this manner will the most lives be saved.

A disaster scene is neither the time nor place to educate and orient people to the medical-disaster plan, medical resources and on-site responsibilities.

If victims are not handled according to a preplanned procedure, the entire medical-care system may become needlessly inundated. Those most familiar with the system's strengths, tolerances and capabilities must assume medical command. Otherwise, those most in need may suffer harmful delays and inappropriate care.

Paramedics and EMTs have an inherent responsibility to provide and coordinate field medical operations at medical disaster scenes. Because EMTs and paramedics arrive during the first few minutes of a disaster, they are initially the highest medical authority on site. The burden of organizing rapid and efficient casualty evacuation rests with them. In a disaster, most of the triage, medical communications and staging areas usually have been established prior to the arrival of the first medical team. In addition, a medical command post and casualty loading areas should be operational. Mobile disaster units also provide additional medical supplies, communications and logistics. Hospital teams may find they are most useful directing medical care and re-triage at the casualty loading areas.

A disaster procedure is dependent upon knowledgeable and cool-headed people taking control and remaining organized. Teamwork and cooperation with other support agencies along the lines of a single pre-established disaster system is absolutely essential.

Following are general guidelines for a medical-disaster plan. They can be used in working closely with participating agencies in coordinating detailed procedures. These medical-disaster procedures are limited to cover medical operations on site at local multi-casualty incidents. These generally include any emergency involving more than 20 victims from transportation accidents, explosions, fires, toxic chemicals, gases, and so on.

EMTs and paramedics will assume initial medical command at such incidents and control triage, treatment, medical communications, supply, medical transportation, manpower assigned to medical operations and coordinate the dispersal of all casualties to medical facilities and casualty collection points. They have the authority to request the activation of the medical-emergency plan and request medical resources as needed.

Depending on the situation, either the fire department or law-enforcement agency is responsible for total incident command. The incident commander has overall responsibility for control and tactical coordination for all public and private agencies at the disaster site. EMTs and paramedics should continue to coordinate their activities with the fire departments in the event incident command is assigned to law enforcement. Upon occurrence of a medical disaster, the first-in EMS unit will establish an ambulance-loading area and use its vehicle as a medical-command post in a safe location. All casualties will be brought to the loading area for re-triage, stabilization and evacuation to medical facilities. If the situation permits, triage will be performed in sectors. However, medical personnel will not enter any dangerous or hazardous environment unless absolutely necessary to save lives. Rescue personnel should perform such functions. Medical personnel can do the most good for the greatest number at the ambulance-loading area. The walking wounded should be separated from the ambulance-loading area to a bus-loading area and monitored by an EMT, paramedic, police officer or firefighter until the Red Cross arrives. They will then be loaded into buses and sent to casualty collection points at the direction of the medical-command post. The dead should not be moved unless directed by the coroner or if they impede lifesaving activities.

The first arriving field personnel will be designated triage officers and will initially serve as the medical commmander. The second initial on-scene field personnel will serve as the medical communications or transportation officer. As soon as additional personnel are on scene, transportation officer functions will be assigned to another paramedic or ambulance supervisor. The triage officer will first perform a medical size-up, estimate the number of casualties and determine what medical resources are needed. The triage officer will then establish a medical-command post and ambulance and bus-loading areas, inform the appropriate person of the medical requirements of the situation and the magnitude of the medical response and advise of the immediate need for certain staging areas. These should be ensured by the incident commmander. The triage officer will control, organize and direct medical operations. Once these logistics are established, the triage officer may engage in triage and supervise all personnel assigned to medical activities. Casualties should be separated and grouped according to their classification.

After a medical size-up is completed, the medical-communications officer will activate the medical-disaster plan and request medical resources. Communication and update with the closest base hospital will immediately follow. The level of medical response and the dispersal of all casualties will be closely coordinated between the controlling hospital and the medical-command post. The medical-command post should also have effective communication with all staging and loading areas.

The medical-transportation officer, designated by the medical commander will supervise the loading of ambulances and their dispatch to area hospitals. Ambulance traffic should be rotated among area hospitals to avoid inadvertently overloading any facility. Updates on receiving capacity should be regularly obtained via the medical-communications officer. Receiving hospitals will expect to receive as many victims as they are capable of handling.

All responding paramedic or ambulance units should report to a staging area as broadcasted. One or two units may be requested to report to the vicinity of the triage area for their manpower, supplies and shelter. These units should park clear of the medical-command post and loading areas and not block transport routes. EMT drivers should stay with their vehicles and not transport patients without direction. Ambulances should rotate through the loading area one or two at a time as directed by the medical-staging officer at the request of the medical-transportation officer.

The paramedic-field supervisor will report to the medical-command post. The field supervisor will first ensure that the disaster procedures are being correctly implemented and EMTs and paramedics are performing their duties properly. The field supervisor may elect to assume medical command at any time from them. Normally, the field supervisor will report to the scene in a disaster-command vehicle equipped with logistic support and medical supplies for 50 casualties.

The fire department is responsible for fire suppression, rescue, extrication, scene safety, medical support, non-medical communications and other functions. The police department is responsible for crowd control, scene security, traffic control including access and egress routes, ambulance and bus-staging operations, disposition of mentally disturbed victims, medical support and other functions.

After all casualties are transported, the medical commander should secure medical operations, and ambulance units should return to normal service as soon as possible.

As soon as practical, but before personnel leave duty at the conclusion of the incident or for their regular shift, a written or tape-recorded statement should be obtained recounting what each individual saw and did on a step-by-step basis. It is necessary to do this while details are fresh in each person's mind. This record will be invaluable in the critique of the incident and may reveal information that necessitates changing the plan.

A P P E N D I X   C

Guidelines for Establishing Ambulance Services

Many states have specific guidelines that they use to evaluate ambulance-service license applications. Although some states license the service to operate in any part of the state, others require separate authorization for each specific service area. The following information was adapted from regulations which guide Missouri's Department of Health in granting ambulance licenses. EMS managers throughout the nation should find this information helpful in considering the viability of any new service area.

When considering a request for licensure of an ambulance service, the Missouri Bureau of Emergency Medical Services employs the following 14-factor analysis in making the difficult decision on whether or not a new service should be licensed. Typically, a convenience and necessity hearing is held to evaluate the 14 criteria. Following the hearing, and upon further review, a formal determination is made on the need for the service.

1. What is the population of the jurisdiction requesting the ambulance service, including tourism and traffic flow through the area? Does the area have a large enough population base to support a new ambulance service?

2. How many calls for service and how many emergency calls are made in the proposed area? What is the average daily rate of calls for this area? Would the area have a large enough demand to maintain a full-time service?

3. What is the average response time for all calls and emergency calls during a recent time period? Is the average response time reasonably prompt or under response-time specifications?

4. What is the quality of existing services and how do the present conditions affect public convenience? Do the nearby ambulance services adequately cover the emergency medical needs of the area? Would a newly licensed ambulance service be an improvement to public convenience?

5. Do mutual-aid ambulance agreements exist among the area under consideration and the nearby ambulance, police, and fire units? Are these agreements necessary for adequate coverage of this particular area?

6. Would the employees of the proposed ambulance service have a sufficient level of clinical experience for maintaining emergency care?

7. Would opportunities exist for personnel to maintain their level of skill? If an additional ambulance service was added, would the dilution of service calls between the ambulance services cause a decay in skills due to inactivity?

8. Are the existing communications capabilities adequate for maintaining medical control and directing paramedics? Would the proposed facilities be an improvement?

9. How will the ambulance service be financed? Are the financial resources available to the proposed ambulance service sufficient for maintaining a full-time service?

10. How will the ambulance service be organized and administered? Does management seem willing to support an ambulance service and is management capable of performing its duties?

11. What will be the total cost of the new ambulance service? Are the benefits that the proposed area would receive worth the expense?

12. Does public opinion in the proposed area favor the establishment of a new ambulance service?

13. Do the local government planning agencies favor establishment of a new ambulance service?

14. Are there any viable alternatives other than licensing a new ambulance service? For example, in some cases volunteer EMTs or firefighters can respond in a non-licensed vehicle and call in an existing service for transport.

Before embarking on a program of licensure, an EMS leader should review the above questions and then objectively decide if there's a legitimate need for an ambulance service in the area.

A P P E N D I X   D

Simplified First Responder Inservice Outline

This is a sample of a training outline that can be adapted for use with your local first-responder organization.

I. Importance and Definition of the First-Responder Role

   A. Stress partnership approach to patient care
      1. show appreciation for past help
      2. reinforce importance of first-responder role (Many patients would not survive without the work that they do.)
      3. stress importance of team approach after EMS arrival

   B. Areas of assistance required at the critical scene
      1. continue life-support functions, if indicated, CPR, ventilation while paramedics do ALS set-up
      2. gather initial information if possible
         a. description of events prior to arrival
         b. patient's medicines and allergies
         c. other pertinent information

   C. Assist with delivery of care
      1. TV set-up
      2. radio set-up
      3. medication set-up
      4. assist with airway or circulation
      5. move patient
      6. obtain additional essential equipment
      7. operate vehicle

II. Specific Equipment

   A. Communications equipment
      1. show APCOR (describe voice or telemetry role—1 watt power)
      2. describe repeater/APCOR relationship
      3. describe set-up of mobile repeater (45 watts of power)
         a. push control
         b. push repeater button
         c. set proper channel
      4. APCOR generally used within three-fourths mile of emergency vehicle in flat, open terrain

   B. IV set-up
      1. show types of IV fluids—show label locations
      2. show how to remove dust cover
      3. show two types drip sets
         a. macro
         b. mini
      4. show extension sets
      5. show aseptic assembly and flush
      6. four or five pieces of 1"-tape helpful
      7. after IV started, hold higher than heart
      8. watch for blood backup and stopped IV

C. Medications
   1. describe and show ampule, bristoject (preload)
   2. show labeling
   3. show assembly of bristoject—have all try
   4. show packages syringes, needles, alcohol preps

D. Advanced airways
   1. show EOA
      a. describe placement in espohagus
      b. explain importance of maintaining mask seal
      c. watch for chest expansion
   2. show endotracheal tube
      a. describe placement in trachea
      b. watch for chest expansion
      c. explain importance of not letting tube move farther in or out
      d. show reference markers on side of tube relative to teeth
      e. hold tube in place

E. Defibrillation
   1. describe safety hazard relative to shock delivered by defibrillator
   2. do not touch patient directly during defibrillation
   3. may hold IV and bag mask without danger
   4. stand up on wet surfaces—do not kneel

F. Moving the arrest patients
   1. if easily accessible, move directly on to cot
   2. if not easily accessible, leave cot outside, move patient on scoop
      or spineboard to cot outside

G. Tour vehicle, show location of essential equipment

A P P E N D I X   E

EMS and Management Information Resources

PART 1 — ASSOCIATIONS AND ORGANIZATIONS

American Ambulance Association
3814 Auburn Blvd., Suite 70
Sacramento, CA 95821
916/483-3827

**American Association for
Respiratory Therapy**
1720 Regal Row, #112
Dallas, TX 75235
214/630-3540

**American Association of Critical-
Care Nurses**
One Civic Plaza
Newport Beach, CA 92660
714/644-9310

**American Board of Emergency
Medicine**
200 Woodland Pass, Suite D
East Lansing, MI 48823
517/332-4800

American Burn Association
1130 E. McDowell Road, Suite B-2
Phoenix, AZ 85006
602/239-2391

**American College of Emergency
Physicians (ACEP)**
P.O. Box 619911
Dallas, TX 75261-9911
214/550-0911

**American College of Healthcare
Executives**
840 North Lake Shore Drive
Chicago, IL 60611
312/943-0544

**American College of Hospital
Administrators (ACHA)**
840 North Lake Shore Drive
Chicago, IL 60611
312/943-0544

**American College of Osteopathic
Emergency Physicians**
5200 South Ellis
Chicago, IL 60615
312/947-2704

**American College of Surgeons
Committee on Trauma**
55 East Erie Street
Chicago, IL 60611
312/664-4050

American Heart Association (AHA)
7320 Greenville Avenue
Dallas, TX 75231
214/750-5300

American Hospital Association
840 North Lake Shore Drive
Chicago, IL 60611
312/280-6000

**American Medical Association
(AMA)**
535 North Dearborn Street
Chicago, IL 60610
312/645-5000

**American Osteopathic Board of
Emergency Medicine**
4150 City Avenue
Philadelphia, PA 19131
215/581-6056

American Red Cross (ARC)
17th and D Streets, NW
Washington, DC 20006
202/737-8300

**American Society for Testing and
Materials (ASTM)**
Committee F-30 on EMS
1916 Race Street
Philadelphia, PA 19103
215/299-5490

American Trauma Society (ATS)
P.O. Box 13526
Baltimore, MD 21203
301/528-6304
800/556-7890

ASHBEAMS
612 Pennsylvania Avenue
San Diego, CA 92103
619/542-0388

Associated Public-Safety
Communications Officers, Inc.
(APCO)
930 Third Avenue
P.O. Box 669
New Smyrna Beach, FL 32070
904/427-3461 or 428-8700

Emergency Care Information
Center
701 Ridgefield Road
Wilton, CT 06897
203/762-3911

Emergency Care Research Institute
(ECRI)
5200 Butler Pike
Plymouth Meeting, PA 19462
215/825/6000

Emergency Medical Service
Institute
5937 Broad Street Mall, Suite 224
Pittsburgh, PA 15206
412/361-3674

Emergency Medicine Foundation
P.O. Box 619911
Dallas, TX 75261-9911
214/550-0911

Emergency Nurses Association (ENA)
666 North Lake Shore Drive,
Suite 1131
Chicago, IL 60611
312/649-0297

Fitch & Associates, Inc.
6812 N.W. Tower Drive
Kansas City, MO 64151-1535
816/741-4422

Helicopter Association
International (HAI)
1619 Duke Street
Alexandria, VA 22314
703/683-4646

International Association of Fire
Chiefs (IAFC)
1329 18th Street, NW
Washington, DC 20036
202/833-3420

International Association of
Firefighters (IAFF)
1750 New York Avenue, NW
Washington, DC 20006
202/737-8484

International Society for Burn
Injuries
2005 Franklin Street
Denver, CO 80205
303/839-1694

JEMS Publishing Company, Inc.
P.O. Box 1026
Solana Beach, CA 92075
619/481-1128

National Association for Search
and Rescue (NASAR)
P.O. Box 50178
Washington, DC 20004
703/352-1349

National Association of EMS
Physicians
190 Lothrop Street
Pittsburgh, PA 15213
803/763-9571

National Association of Emergency
Medical Technicians (NAEMT)
9140 Ward Parkway
Kansas City, MO 64114
816/444-3500

National Association of State EMS
Directors (NASEMSD)
Dept. of Health and Welfare
Statehouse
Boise, ID 83720
208/334-4245

National Council of State EMS
Training Coordinators (NCSEMSTC)
P.O. Box 3824
Pojoaque, NM 87501-0824
505/827-2509

National EMS Pilot's Association
(AirNet)
P.O. Box 2354
Pearland, TX 77588
713/997-2563

National Fire Protection
Association (NFPA)
Batterymarch Park
Quincy, MA 02269
617/770-3000

National Flight Paramedic
Association
800 East Dawson
Tyler, TX 75701
214/531-4945

**National Flight Nurses Association
(NFNA)**
P.O. Box 8222
Rapid City, SD 57709
605/343-4464

**National Registry of EMTs
(NREMT)**
P.O. Box 29233
Columbus, OH 43229
614/888-4484

National Safety Council
444 North Michigan Avenue
Chicago, IL 60611
312/527-4800

**National Spinal Cord Injury
Hotline**
2201 Argonne Drive
Baltimore, MD 21218
800/526-3456
800/638-1733 (in MD)

**National Study Center for Trauma
and EMS**
UMBC TF-142
Baltimore, MD 21228
301/455-3666

**Society of Teachers of Emergency
Medicine (STEM)**
P.O. Box 619911
Dallas, TX 75261-9911
214/550-0921

**University Association for
Emergency Medicine**
900 West Ottawa
Lansing, MI 48915
517/485-5484

PART 2 — GOVERNMENT AGENCIES

Dept. of Transportation
EMS Division, Room 6124
400 7th St., S.W.
Washington, D.C. 20590
202/366-5440

**Environmental Protection Agency
(EPA)**
Public Information Center
820 Quincy Street, NW
Washington, DC 20011
202/829-3535

**Federal Communications
Commission (FCC)**
1919 M Street, NW
Washington, DC 20554
202/632-7000

**FEMA
U.S. Fire Administration**
16825 South Seton Avenue
Emmitsburg, MD 21727
301/447-1000

**Health Care Finance
Administration**
6325 Security Blvd.,
Room 700 E. High Rise
Baltimore, MD 21207
301/594-7914

**National Emergency Training
Center**
Learning Resource Center
16825 South Seton Avenue
Emmitsburg, MD 21727
301/447-1032
800/638-1821

National Fire Academy
16825 South Seton Avenue
Emmitsburg, MD 21727
301/447-1000

**Occupational Safety and Health
Administration (OSHA)**
Department of Labor
3rd St. and Constitution Ave., NW
Washington DC 20210
202/523-8148

PART 3 — SELECTED FEDERAL
HEALTH INFORMATION CLEARINGHOUSES

Cancer Information Clearinghouse
National Cancer Institute
9000 Rockville Pike
Bldg. 31, Room 10A-18
Bethesda, MD 20892
301/496-5583

**Center for Health Promotion and
Education Centers for Disease
Control**
1600 Clifton Road, NE
Bldg. 1 South, Room SSB249
Atlanta, GA 30333
404/329-3492

**Clearinghouse for Occupational
Safety and Health Information**
Technical Info. Branch
4676 Columbia Parkway
Cincinnati, OH 45226
513/533-8326

**Clearinghouse on Child Abuse and
Neglect Information**
P.O. Box 1182
Washington, DC 20013
301/251-5157

**Clearinghouse on Health Indexes
National Center for Health
Statistics**
Office of Analysis and
Epidemiology Programs
3700 East-West Highway
Room 2-27
Hyattsville, MD 20782
301/436-7035

**Consumer Product Safety
Commission**
Washington, DC 20013
800/638-2772

**High Blood Pressure Information
Center**
National Institutes of Health (NIH)
9000 Rockville Pike
Bethesda, MD 20892
301/496-1809

**National Clearinghouse for Alcohol
Information (NCALI)**
P.O. Box 2345
Rockville, MD 20852
301/468-2600

**National Clearinghouse for Drug
Abuse Information**
P.O. Bos 416
Kensington, MD 20795
301/443-6500

**National Diabetes Information
Clearinghouse**
Box NDIC
Bethesda, MD 20892
301/468-2162

**National Injury Information
Clearinghouse**
5401 Westbard Avenue, Room 625
Washington, DC 20207
301/492-6424

**National Institute of Mental Health
Public Inquiries Branch**
5600 Fishers Lane, Room 15C-05
Rockville, MD 20857
301/443-4513

**National Rehabilitation
Information Center**
4407 Eighth Street, NE
Washington, DC 20017
202/635-5826
800/34-NARIC

**National Sudden Infant Death
Syndrome/Primary Care**
8201 Greensboro Drive
Suite 600
McLean, VA 22102
703/821-8955

ODPHP Health Information Center
P.O. Box 1133
Washington, DC 20013-1133
202/429-9091 (in DC)
800/336-4797

**U.S. Consumer Product Safety
Commission**
Washington, DC 20207

PART 4 — SUGGESTED READINGS
IN MANAGEMENT AND LEADERSHIP

Argyris, Chris; *Human Behavior in Organizations* (Harper and Row, New York, 1957)

Blake, R.R., and Mouton, J.S.; *The Managerial Grid* (Gulf Publishing Co., Texas, 1964)

Bennis, Warren G.; *Changing Organizations* (McGraw Hill, New York, 1966)

Dernocoeur, Kate B.; *Streetsense—Communication, Safety and Control* (Brady, 1985)

Fournies, Ferdnand F.; *Coaching for Improved Work Performance* (Van Nostrand Reinhold Co., New York, 1978)

Gibb, Jack R.; *Trust: A New View of Personal and Organizational Effectiveness* (Guild of Tutors Press, Los Angeles, 1978)

Hersey, Paul, and Blanchard, Kenneth H.; *Management of Organizational Behavior: Utilizing Human Resources* (Prentice-Hall, Englewood Cliffs, N.J., 1982)

Herzberg, Frederick, Mausner, B., and Snyderman, B.B.; *The Motivation to Work* (John Wiley and Sons, New York, 1959)

Kanter, Rosabeth Moss; *The Change Masters* (Simon and Schuster, New York, 1983)

Lakein, Alan; *How to Get Control of Your Time and Your Life* (Signet, New York, 1973)

Lane, Byron D.; *Managing People* (Oasis Press, Sunnyvale, CA., 1985)

Maslow, A.H.; *Motivation and Personality* (Harper and Row, New York, 1954)

McGregor, Douglas; *The Human Side of Enterprise* (McGraw Hill, New York, 1960)

Naisbitt, John; *Megatrends* (Warner Books, New York, 1982)

Naisbitt, John, and Aburdene, Patricia; *Re-inventing the Corporation* (Warner Books, New York, 1985)

Odiorne, George S.; *Management by Objectives* (Pitman Publishing, New York, 1965)

Ouchi, William G.; *Theory Z: How American Business Can Meet the Japanese Challenge* (Addison-Wesley, Mass., 1980)

Peters, Thomas J., and Waterman, Robert H. Jr.; *In Search of Excellence* (Harper and Row, New York, 1982)

Peters, Tom, and Austin, Nancy; *A Passion for Excellence: The Leadership Difference* (Random House, New York, 1985)

Rogers, Carl; *Freedom to Learn* (Charles E. Merrill, Columbus, OH, 1969)

Simmons, John, and Mares, William; *Working Together* (Alfred E. Knopf, New York, 1983)

Toffler, Alvin; *The Third Wave* (Bantam Books, New York, 1981)

A P P E N D I X F

State EMS Offices

For information about EMS training, regulations and related subjects in a given state, the best bet is to contact the lead EMS agency in that state.

Alabama
State of Alabama Dept. of Health
Emergency Medical Svcs. Div.
State Office Bldg., Rm. 644
Montgomery, AL 36130-1701
205/261-5261

Alaska
Emergency Medical Svcs. Section
Dept. of Health & Social Svcs.
P.O. Box H-06C
Juneau, AK 99811
907/465-3027

Arizona
Div. of EMS & Health Care
Facilities
Arizona Dept. of Health Services
411 North 24th Street
Phoenix, AZ 85008
602/220-6400

Arkansas
Office Emergency Medical Svcs.
Arkansas Dept. of Health
4815 W. Markham Street
Little Rock, AR 72205-3867
501/661-2262

California
Emergency Medical Svcs.
Authority
1600 9th Street, Rm. 400
Sacramento, CA 95814
916/322-4336

Colorado
Emergency Medical Svcs. Div.
Colorado Department of Health
4210 E. 11th Avenue
Denver, CO 80220
313/331-4915

Connecticut
Office of Emergency Medical Svcs.
Dept. of Health
150 Washington Street
Hartford, CT 06106
203/566-7336

Delaware
Emergency Medical Svcs.
Capitol Square
Jesse S. Cooper Memorial Bldg.
Dover, DE 19901
302/736-4710

District of Columbia
Emergency Health & Medical Svcs.
Dept. of Human Services
1875 Connecticut Ave., N.W.,
Rm. 833-D
Washington, DC 20009
202/673-6744

Florida
Emergency Medical Svcs.
Dept. of Health & Rehabilitation
1317 Winewood Blvd., PDHEMS
Tallahassee, FL 32301
904/487-1911

Georgia
Emergency Medical Svcs. Office
State Dept. of Human Resources
878 Peachtree St., N.E., Rm. 207
Atlanta, GA 30309
404/894-6505

Guam
Office of EMS, Dept. of Public
Health and Social Svcs.
P.O. Box 2816
Agana, Guam 96910
671/734-2783/2951, ext. 202/206

Hawaii
EMSS Br. State of Hawaii
Dept. of Health
3627 Kilauea Ave., Rm. 102
Honolulu, HI 96816
808/735-5267

Idaho
Emergency Medical Svcs. Bureau
Dept. of Health & Welfare
450 W. State Street
Boise, ID 83720
208/334-5994

Illinois
Div. of Emergency Medical Svcs.
and Highway Safety
Illinois Dept. of Public Health
525 W. Jefferson St., Rm. 450
Springfield, IL 62761
217/785-2080

Indiana
Indiana EMS Commission
State Office Bldg., Rm. 315
100 N. Senate Avenue
Indianapolis, IN 46204
317/232-3980

Iowa
Emergency Medical Svcs.
Iowa Dept. of Public Health
Lucas State Office Building
Des Moines, IA 50319-0075
515/281-3741

Kansas
Bureau of Emergency Medical Svcs.
Dept. of Highway and Patrol
111 West 6th Street
Topeka, KS 66603
913/296-7296

Kentucky
Emergency Medical Svcs.
Cabinet for Human Resources
275 E. Main Street
Frankfort, KY 40621
502/564-8963

Louisiana
Bureau of Emergency Medical Svcs.
200 Lafayette Street, Suite 600
Baton Rouge, LA 70801
504/342-2600

Maine
Maine Emergency Medical Svcs.
295 Water Street
Augusta, ME 04330
207/298-3953

Maryland
EMS Field Operations
31 S. Greene Street
Baltimore, MD 21201
301/528-3160

Emergency Medical Svcs.—MIEMSS
22 S. Greene Street
Baltimore, MD 21201
301/528-5085

Massachusetts
Office of Emergency Medical Svcs.
Dept. of Public Health
80 Boylston St., Suite 1040
Boston, MA 02116
617/451-3433

Michigan
Div. of Emergency Medical Svcs.
3500 N. Logan
P.O. Box 30035
Lansing, MI 48909
517/335-8503

Minnesota
EMS Section, Dept. of Health
717 Delaware Street, S.E.
P.O. Box 9441
Minneapolis, MN 55440
612/623-5284

Mississippi
Office of Emergency Medical Svcs.
State Board of Health
P.O. Box 1700
Jackson, MS 39215
601/354-7075

Missouri
Bureau of Emergency Medical Svcs.
Missouri Dept. of Health
P.O. Box 570
Jefferson City, MO 65102
314/751-4022

Montana
Emergency Medical Svcs. Bureau
Dept. of Health & Env. Sciences
Cogswell Building
Helena, MT 59620
406/444-3895

Nebraska
Div. of Emergency Medical Svcs.
301 Centennial Mall S., 3rd Fl.
Box 95007
Lincoln, NE 68509-5007
402/471-2158

Nevada
Emergency Medical Svcs. Office
505 E. King Street
Capitol Complex, Kinkead Bldg.
Carson City, NV 89710
702/885-3065

New Hampshire
Emergency Medical Svcs.
Health & Welfare Building
Hazen Drive
Concord, NH 03301
603/271-4569

New Jersey
Director, Emergency Medical Svcs.
State Dept. of Health
C.N. 363
Trenton, NJ 08625
609/292-0782

Emergency Care Monitoring
Emergency Medical Svcs.
State Dept. of Health
C.N. 363
Trenton, NJ 08625
609/292-0782

New Mexico
Primary Care & EMS Bureau
Health Services Division
Health & Environment Dept.
P.O. Box 968
Santa Fe, NM 87504-0968
505/827-2509

New York
Emergency Medical Svcs.
Development Program
ESP Tower Building, Rm. 2270
22nd Floor, Empire State Plaza
Albany, NY 12237
518/474-3171

North Carolina
Office of Emergency Medical Svcs.
701 Barbour Drive
Raleigh, NC 27603
919/733-2285

North Dakota
Emergency Health Services Div.
Dept. of Health
State Capitol Building
Bismarck, ND 58505
701/224-2388

Ohio
Dept. of Public Safety Services
65 S. Front Street, Rm. 918
Columbus, OH 43215
614/344-0331, ext. 205

Training and Certification
Dept. of Public Safety Services
65 S. Front Street, Rm. 918
Columbus, OH 43215
614/466-9447

Oklahoma
Emergency Medical Svcs.
1000 N.E. 10th, Rm. 211
P.O. Box 53551
Oklahoma City, OK 73152
405/271-4062

Oregon
Emergency Medical Svcs.
State Health Department
P.O. Box 231
Portland, OR 97201
503/229-6365

Pennsylvania
Division of Emergency Medical
Health Svcs.
Pennsylvania Dept. of Health
P.O. Box 90, Rm. 1033
Health & Welfare Building
Harrisburg, PA 17108
717/787-8741

Puerto Rico
Emergency Medical Svcs.
G.P.O. Box 71423
San Juan, Puerto Rico 00936
809/753-4244

Rhode Island
Div. of Emergency Medical Svcs.
Dept. of Health
75 Davis Street
Providence, RI 02908
401/277-2401

South Carolina
Div. of Emergency Medical Svcs.
Dept. of Health & Environment
Control
2600 Bull Street
Columbia, SC 29201
803/737-7009

South Dakota
Emergency Medical Svcs. Program
Dept. of Health
Joe Foss Building
523 E. Capitol Street
Pierre, SD 57501
605/773-3737

Tennessee
Tennessee Dept. of Health & Env.
Div. of Emergency Medical Svcs.
283 Plus Park Boulevard
Nashville, TN 37217
615/367-6278

Texas
EMS Division
Texas Dept. of Health
1100 W. 49th Street
Austin, TX 78756
512/465-2601

Utah
Bureau of Emergency
Medical Svcs.
P.O. Box 16660
Salt Lake City, UT 84116-0660
801/538-6435

Vermont
Emergency Medical Svcs. Div.
Box 70, 60 Main Street
Burlington, VT 05402
802/863-7310

Virgin Islands
Emergency Medical Svcs.
Dept. of Health
P.O. Box 7309
St. Thomas, Virgin Islands 00801
809/774-9000, ext. 316

Virginia
Bureau of Emergency
Medical Svcs.
State Dept. of Health
109 Governor Street, Rm. 1001
Richmond, VA 23219
804/786-5188

Washington
Emergency Medical Svcs.
Health Services Division
DSHS Mail Stop ET-34
Olympia, WA 98504
206/753-5898/2095

West Virginia
Emergency Medical Svcs.
Dept. of Health
Building 3, Rm. 426
1800 Washington Street, East
East Charleston, WV 25305
304/348-3956

Wisconsin
Emergency Medical Svcs. Section
Division of Health
Box 309
Madison, WI 53701
608/266-1568

Wyoming
Emergency Medical Svcs. Program
Hathaway Building, Rm. 527
Cheyenne, WY 82002
307/777-7955

A   P   P   E   N   D   I   X   G

EMS Salary Survey

JEMS, the Journal of Emergency Medical Services, published its first national EMS salary survey in January 1982. The survey has been conducted periodically ever since, with the last survey published in January 1985. Most recently, *JEMS* and the people at Fitch & Associates teamed up to conduct a 1987 salary survey. The information for the salary was gathered in the summer of 1987. The data was compiled by an independent research firm, Scott Gard and Associates, with offices in Kansas City, Missouri and Washington, D.C.

THE SURVEY SAMPLE

JEMS recognized that the surveying methodology needed to be improved to provide the most reliable statistics to the EMS industry. Declines of the average salary in four of five job classifications between the 1984 and 1985 surveys indicated that the respondents from year to year may vary significantly and lead to results which may not reflect actual trends and situations. It is unlikely that EMTs, EMT-Ps, dispatchers and supervisors actually experienced reductions in annual salaries during 1984.

To address this anomaly, we developed a method to standardize the way information is obtained. Over 200 organizations were selected to provide a wide range of types of services (for example, fire department, private or hospital-based), size of services and locations. These services were contacted individually and asked to participate in the survey process. One hundred sixty-seven agreed to participate in this and future surveys. The same services will again be providing information for the survey in 1988, providing a "Dow Jones" for the ambulance industry.

The first year will provide a baseline against which changes and trends can be demonstrated in the future. Each extensive survey dictated 485 data inputs with 187 separate question items.

The total number of respondents for this advance analysis is 111. This represents a significant increase in participation over previous surveys. With the agreement of these services to continue participation, annual survey results should provide valuable information for ambulance service providers.

Breakdown of information is in three major areas: type of service, region and population served. While the focus of the project concentrated on the salary results, other information emerged and will be reported in *JEMS*.

Figure F-1 shows the breakdown of services by type of provider. All 111 respondents answered the question. Eighteen percent of those responding are private providers, 68 percent are public providers, 22 percent are hospital based. Three percent represent other non-profit operations. This represents a shift from the 1985 survey, with a much larger percentage of response coming from public-sector organizations, particularly fire departments.

This year the country was divided into four regions in order to provide a larger sample from each area. Figure F-2 lists the number of respondents and percentage of type for each region. Four services did not indicate the state in which they operate.

Seventy-one percent of the respondents serve a primary service area with the population range of 100,000 to 1,000,000. The distribution of services by the size population served is presented in Figure F-3.

ANNUAL COMPENSATION

This year's survey defined each position by function and responsibility. This was done to differentiate between some middle-management positions and to compare public service (for example, fire department) positions with other sectors and types of providers. Thirteen separate positions were defined, and nine are included here for comparison in Figure F-4.

The questionnaire specifically asked for the average salary for each position within the organization. For analysis, the means of these salary averages were calculated. Using the mean instead of the direct average levels the effect of extremely low or extremely high salaries within each category. The number of respondents within each category is included in the total average salaries.

Figure F-4 presents the information on average salaries for various types of providers. These figures represent a significant increase from the salaries examined in the 1985 survey. The 1985 survey was based on information compiled in 1984. This analysis is based upon 1987 information. The difference in methodology of information accumulation could also be responsible for the changes. The increase in responses from the public sector also shifts the overall averages upward. Fire departments lead in compensation for all positions identified in the survey.

Comparisons between the 1987 and the 1985 (1984 information) results demonstrate the following increases:

	1987	1985	% Change
Paramedics			
Overall	24,250	18,540	+ 30.8%
Private	21,530	16,721	+ 28.8%
F.D.	29,060	20,706	+ 40.3%
EMTs			
Overall	18,710	14,520	+ 28.9%
Private	15,690	12,754	+ 23.0%
F.D.	26,110	18,818	+ 38.3%
EMT-Is			
Overall	18,830	14,716	+ 28.0%
Private	17,780	13,881	+ 28.1%
F.D.	26,110	25,528	+ 2.3%
Dispatcher			
Overall	18,710	15,589	+ 20.0%
Private	18,170	14,100	+ 28.9%
F.D.	24,260	22,007	+ 10.2%

Other categories in Figure F-4 did not have comparable positions presented in the 1985 survey. Dramatic increases are represented in the comparisons. This lends itself to multiple explanations. Increased competition for qualified personnel could cause such an increase. Many areas have experienced difficulty in attracting and maintaining ambulance personnel. Undercompensation for ambulance personnel three years ago could also explain part of the increases.

Due to the small size of the sample, the significance and accuracy compared to the actual national average cannot be stated. The purpose of this survey is primarily to establish a base against which comparisons can be made in future surveys.

OTHER INFORMATION

A variety of information was compiled and analyzed from the survey, and some of the significant highlights are included in this section. One question asks if the service typically provides transportation for the patient from the scene. All of the private services responding to the survey provide transportation while 71 percent of the public services offer transportation. Ninety-three percent of all services polled respond to all requests received by dispatch. Seven percent, and 10 percent of the fire departments, do not respond to all requests.

Half of the respondents use some type of medical dispatch priority system and 57 percent differentiate between ALS and BLS in their response classification. Fifty-six percent of all services (76.5 percent of the privates and 53.7 percent of the fire departments) typically provide pre-arrival instructions to callers. Of those which provide pre-arrival instructions only 38 percent use pre-arrival instruction cards and 56 percent allow the dispatchers to independently improvise pre-arrival instructions.

Finally, the levels of training for dispatchers vary considerably.

EMT only	34.2%
EMT-P	5.4%
Medical Dispatch Course	22.5%
No Special Training	37.8%

Eighty-six percent of the services indicated that they had some type of physician medical control or advice, with 74 percent paying for physician services.

FIGURE F-1: Sample Group

	No. of Respondents	Percentage
Private	18	16.22%
Public		
Fire dept.	42	37.84%
Third service	12	10.81%
Other public	14	12.61%
Hospital	22	19.82%
Other NFP	3	2.70%
Total	111	100.00%

FIGURE F-2: Geographic Distribution of Respondents

Region	No. of Respondents	Percentage
North-Eastern Connecticut, Maine, Massachusetts, New Hampshire, Delaware, New Jersey, New York, Pennsylvania, Rhode Island, Vermont, Michigan	11	10.28%
Western Alaska, Arizona, California, Hawaii, Idaho, Nevada, New Mexico, Oregon, Utah, Washington, Colorado, Texas, Montana, Wyoming	48	44.86%
Central North Dakota, South Dakota, Nebraska, Kansas, Oklahoma, Ohio, Minnesota, Iowa, Missouri, Illinois, Wisconsin, Indiana	21	19.63%
South-Eastern Florida, Georgia, Alabama, Mississippi, Arkansas, Tennessee, North Carolina, South Carolina, Kentucky, Virginia, West Virginia, Louisiana, Maryland	27	25.23%
Total	107	100.00%

FIGURE F-3: Population Served

Population Range	Respondents	Percentage
Less than 20,000	10	9.09%
20,000 to 49,999	6	5.45%
50,000 to 99,999	11	10.00%
100,000 to 249,999	32	29.09%
250,000 to 999,999	39	35.45%
Greater than 1,000,000	12	10.91%
Total	110	100.00%

FIGURE F-4: Annual Compensation

Provider Type	Executive Director	Admin. Director	Operations Manager	Div./Ops. Supervisor	Field Supervisor	Paramedic	EMT Intermediate	EMT-Basic	Dispatcher
Private	46,500	36,400	30,180	27,750	23,870	21,530	17,780	15,690	18,170
Public	45,630	41,250	42,280	36,660	31,620	26,620	23,210	22,640	22,290
Fire dept.	51,930	49,300	49,920	42,450	35,790	29,060	26,110	26,110	24,260
Third serv.	45,000	35,170	34,270	26,880	24,890	23,090	19,000	18,140	20,860
Other pub.	27,250	34,090	29,800	25,500	23,500	21,400	16,500	15,170	18,250
Hospital	36,000	32,220	27,090	25,500	24,000	20,400	16,000	14,060	16,570
Other NFP	37,000	n/a	22,500	20,000	22,500	23,000	8,500	n/a	11,000
Mean Salary	42,470	38,930	37,210	34,260	28,510	24,250	18,830	18,710	20,230

A P P E N D I X   H

Sample Chart of Accounts

ACCT. #	CROSS REF.	ACCOUNT
		Support/Revenue
401	_____	Fees from Patients (ALS)
402	_____	Fees from Patients (BLS)
403	_____	Fees from Patients (Wheelchair)
405	_____	Adjustments
406	_____	Allowance for Bad Debt
407	_____	Contractual Allowance
408	_____	Fees (Special Events)
409	_____	Fees from Governmental Agencies
411	_____	Fees from Other Organizations
412	_____	Collection on Accts. Previously Charged Off
413	_____	Gain on Sale of Assets
414	_____	Other Sales
415	_____	Other Income
416	_____	Gifts/Bequests/Contributions
		Expenditures
501	_____	Salaries & Wages--Administrative/Support
502	_____	Salaries & Wages--Production
511	_____	Employee Group Insurance
512	_____	Retirement Plan
521	_____	Payroll Taxes--Social Security (FICA)
522	_____	State Unemployment Insurance (SUI)
523	_____	Federal Unemployment (FUTA)
524	_____	Workman's Compensation

Chart of Accounts   Page 2

525	_____	Uniforms
526	_____	Tuition/Training
531	_____	Professional Services--Legal
532	_____	Professional Services--Audit & Accounting
533	_____	Professional Services--General
535	_____	Contractual Services--Aircraft Lease
536	_____	Contractual Services--Flight Hr. Charges
541	_____	Office Supplies
542	_____	Office Equipment--Purchased
543	_____	Office Equipment--Rent/Lease
544	_____	Office Equipment--Maintenance
545	_____	Medical Supplies
546	_____	Medical Equipment--Purchased
547	_____	Medical Equipment--Rent/Lease
548	_____	Medical Equipment--Maintenance
549	_____	Laundry
551	_____	Vehicles--Insurance
552	_____	Vehicles--License & Taxes
553	_____	Vehicles--Gasoline & Oil
554	_____	Vehicles--Tires
555	_____	Vehicles--Rent/Lease
556	_____	Vehicles--Maintenance
557	_____	Aero Fuel
558	_____	Small Tools
561	_____	Occupancy
562	_____	Utilities
563	_____	Facilities--Improvements
564	_____	Facilities--Maintenance

Chart of Accounts   Page 3

565	_____	Facilities--Equipment
571	_____	Telephone--Fixed Monthly Charges
572	_____	Telephone--Variable/Toll Charges
581	_____	Postage
582	_____	Shipping
591	_____	Communications Equipment--Purchases
592	_____	Communications Equipment--Rent/Lease
593	_____	Communications Equipment--Maintenance
611	_____	Printing & Artwork
621	_____	Public Information & Education
622	_____	Employee/Community Relations
623	_____	Marketing & Advertising
624	_____	Recruiting
625	_____	Dues & Subscriptions
631	_____	Insurance--Liability & Surety Bonds
632	_____	Insurance--All Risk & Equipment Property Floaters
633	_____	Taxes & Licenses
634	_____	Service Charges
635	_____	Administrative--Miscellaneous
636	_____	Charity & Donation Expenses
641	_____	Travel--Administrative
642	_____	Travel--Production
651	_____	Collection Expense
701	_____	Interest Expense
711	_____	Depreciation
721	_____	Amortization of Covenants
731	_____	Management Fee

A P P E N D I X   I

Sample Run Report

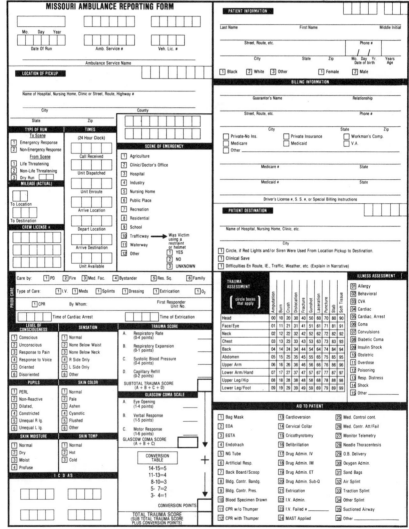

MISSOURI DIVISION OF HEALTH, BUREAU OF EMERGENCY MEDICAL SERVICES

Appendix I (continued)

PATIENT AUTHORIZATION & RELEASE

I, the undersigned, hereby authorize payment directly to the ambulance service shown on the left, benefits otherwise payable to me but not to exceed the regular charges for this type of service. If I am entitled to Medicare benefits, I authorize any holder of medical or other information about me to release to Social Security Administration or its intermediaries or carriers, any information needed for this or related Medicare claim. I permit a copy of this authorization to be used in place of the original, and request payment of medical insurance benefits either to myself or to the party who accepts assignments below. I understand I am financially responsible to the ambulance service listed above for charges not covered by this authorization and do hereby guarantee payment of this bill within forty-five (45) days. I further agree that if collection is made by suit or otherwise, I agree to pay all collection costs including a reasonable attorney's fee. I hereby approve release of information pertinent to hospital confinement, doctor's treatment, and diagnosis for claims for insurance benefits. NOTE: Nothing in the above statement shall provide a basis for denial of either emergency care or emergency transport because of inability to pay.

Signed X _____ Patient or Policy Holder

How Was Patient Found/Mechanism of Injury:	Med Hx:
Chief Complaint	Med Alert: ☐ Tag ☐ Card Dx:
	Rx Meds:
	Allergies:
Duration:	Personal Physician:

TIME	BLOOD PRESSURE	PULSE	RESPIRATION
	/ ☐ Auscultation ☐ Palpation	☐ Regular ☐ Thready ☐ Bounding ☐ Irregular ☐ Weak	☐ Rales ☐ Wheezes ☐ Ronchi ☐ Clear
	/ ☐ Auscultation ☐ Palpation	☐ Regular ☐ Thready ☐ Bounding ☐ Irregular ☐ Weak	☐ Rales ☐ Wheezes ☐ Ronchi ☐ Clear
	/ ☐ Auscultation ☐ Palpation	☐ Regular ☐ Thready ☐ Bounding ☐ Irregular ☐ Weak	☐ Rales ☐ Wheezes ☐ Ronchi ☐ Clear

ON SCENE COMMUNICATIONS: ☐ Radio ☐ Telephone ☐ None ☐ Other _____

MEDICAL CONTROL RECEIVED FROM: _____

Name of Physician or Nurse   Name of Hospital

NARRATIVE SHOULD INCLUDE A COMPLETE CHRONOLOGICAL FLOW OF EVENTS, INCLUDING TIMES, PATIENT CONDITION, EACH PROCEDURE RENDERED AND HOW EACH PROCEDURE AFFECTED THE PATIENT'S CONDITION. IF PATIENT IS MONITORED, DESCRIBE ECG AND STAPLE ECG STRIP TO ORIGINAL FORM.

☐ Check, if review by medical advisor is requested

Signature of Person Receiving Patient   Signature of Crew

MISSOURI BUREAU OF EMS COPY

A P P E N D I X   J

Procedures for Vehicle Equipment and Preventive Maintenance

Courtesy Medevac Midamerica, Inc.

PREVENTIVE MAINTENANCE RECORD

Date	Unit Number	Year	Make	Vehicle ID No.	Preventive Maintenance A B C D E	Division	Mileage

A Check 3,000 Miles or One (1) Mo.

- Oil Change G/D/LP* .... No/Yes
- Oil Filter G/D/LP* .... No/Yes
- Fuel Filter G/D/LP* .... No/Yes
- Air Cleaner .... Good/Replace
- Power Steering .... Full/Add
- Anti-Freeze (Degree of Protection) ____°
- Brake Fluid .... Full/Add
- Emergency Brake .... Good/Repair
- Wiper & Blades .... Good/Replace
- Window Washer Fluid .... Full/Add
- Transmission Fluid .... Full/Add
- Differential Fluid .... Full/Add
- Belts .... Good/Worn/Loose
- Hoses .... Good/Replace
- Heater Cond. Front .... Good/Repair
-              Rear .... Good/Repair
- Defroster Condition .... Good/Repair
- A/C Cond. Front .... Good/Repair
-            Rear .... Good/Repair
- Jack Vehicle Up .... No/Yes
- Grease Chassis & Drive Shaft ..... No/Yes
- Check Alignment .... Good/Bad
- Check for Leaky Shocks .... No/Yes
- Check for Broken Springs .... No/Yes
- Emergency Lights .... Good/Repair
- Vehicle Lights .... Good/Repair
- Fog Lights .... Good/Repair
- Spot Lights Right .... Good/Repair
-              Left .... Good/Repair
- Siren .... Good/Repair
- Alternating Head Lights .... Good/Repair
- Check All Glow Plugs Good/Repair #____
- Voltage Monitor .... Good/Repair
- Throttle Set @ _____ RPM
- Check All Gauges .... Good/Repair
- Check Vehicle Horn .... Good/Repair
- Check Air Horn .... Good/Repair
- Check Exhaust System for Noise and Leaks ... Good/Replace
- Torque Lug Nuts .... No/Yes

Battery Test Sun VAT 40:   (A Check)

- Right Battery (1) .... Good/Bad
  (250 Draw at 20 sec. > 10.4 Volts)
- Left Battery (2) .... Good/Bad
- Alternator Output .... _____ Amp
- Starter Draw .... _____ Amp
- Regulator Max. Voltage .... _____ Volts
- Clean Battery Terminals .... No/Yes

Tires: (A Check)

Tire Air PSI	Front	___ / ___ /
(Measure Tire	Single	___ / ___ /
Wear in 32nds)	Duals	___ / ___ /

EXAMPLE: 13/32nds Wear / 50 PSI

A-Check Cont'd.:

- Check Failsafe Box .... No/Yes
- Lubricate All Door Hinges .... No/Yes
- Check All Mirrors .... Good/Replace
- Check All Glass .... Good/Replace
- Check Oil Dipstick .... No/Yes

* G Gas   D. Diesel   LP-Propane

Problems Found, Comments:

_____

_____

B Check   12,000 Miles

- Do All of A-Check .... No/Yes
- Replace All Belts .... No/Yes
- Level Failsafe Box .... No/Yes

C Check   18,000 Miles

- Do All of A-Check .... No/Yes
- Remove All Wheels and Inspect Brakes ... No/Yes
- Clean Wheel Bearings & Inspect ... No/Yes
- Balanced All Tires .... No/Yes
- Tune Up: Gas, LP .... No/Yes
- Drain Transmission and Replace Fluid & Filters ... No/Yes

D Check   24,000 Miles

- Do All of A-Check .... No/Yes
- Replace All belts .... No/Yes
- Level Failsafe Box .... No/Yes

E Check   36,000 Miles

- Do All of A, B & C-Check .... No/Yes
- Drain Differential and Replace Fluid ... No/Yes
- Replace All Hoses .... No/Yes
- Replace Thermostat .... No/Yes
- Replace All Shocks .... No/Yes

DIESEL:

- Remove All Injection and Clean & Check for Leaks Test ... No/Yes
- Adjustment of Timing .... No/Yes

Work Done By _____

Road Tested By _____

Appendix J (continued)

5323

WORK ORDER

MEDEVAC

| Date | Unit Number | Year | Make | Vehicle ID No. | Preventive Maintenance A B C D E | Equip. Failure # | Accident | Mileage | Gas Diesel Petroleum |

Division

| Code | REPAIR DESCRIPTION | Hrs. | Cost |

| Code | Quan. | Part Number | Description | Unit Price | Extended Price |

00 Accidents
10 Body/Cab Misc.
11 Glass/Mirrors
12 Wipers/Blades
13 AM/FM Radio
14 Heater Front/Rear
15 Defroster
16 Air Cond. Front/Rear
17 Seats and Seat Belts
18 Door and Hinges

20 Chassis/Misc.
21 Brakes
22 Emergency Brakes
23 Springs
24 Shocks
25 Steering
26 Alignment
27 Wheels
28 Tires

30 Cooling/Misc.
31 Water Pump
32 Radiator
33 Hoses Radiator/Heater
34 Belts

40 Electrical/Misc.
41 Alternator
42 Regulator
43 Starter
44 Battery L/R
45 Turn Signals L/R
46 Brake Lights
47 Hazard Lights
48 Back Up Lights
49 Headlights Hi/Lo
50 Headlight Flasher
51 Fog Lights
52 Spot Lights L/R
53 Light Bar
54 Strobe Emer. Light
55 Cowl Beacons
56 Scene Lts. L/R/Rear
57 Auto Throttle
58 Siren W.y./h-l. pa. elec. air manual, radio spk

59 Horn
60 Air Horn
61 Int. Lights Hi-Lo
    Dome/Att. Panel
62 Suction/Rear Vent
70 Shore Line
71 110 Vac. Recp.
    Interior/PDQ Panel
72 110 Heater/Batt. Cond
73 GFCI On/Off Trip

80 Drive Train/Misc.
81 Transmission
82 Drive Shaft
83 Differential
84 Rear Axles
90 Engine/Misc. G/D/LP
    PM
91 Idle Smooth/Rough
92 Exhaust Misc./Leak
93 Mufflers
94 Glow Plugs
95 Injection
97 Injection Pump

100 Vehicle Radios
200 On-Board Equipment

Total Labor

Owner Name _____
Address _____
City _____ State _____ Zip _____
Contact _____ Phone _____

Work Done By _____
Road Tested By _____
Sublet Repair _____
Vendor _____
P. O. # _____
Total Sublet _____

Total Parts _____
Sublet Cost _____
Labor Cost _____
BOTTOM LINE _____

© 1986 MEDEVAC, INC.

A P P E N D I X   K

Index

About The Authors

Joseph J. Fitch, Ph.D., is a former paramedic whose career led him to become a successful entrepreneur, organizational development expert and consultant. One of the first paramedics trained in the United States, Dr. Fitch's EMS experience includes leadership roles in major private and public ambulance services. As president of Fitch & Associates, he leads a successful consulting team in its assignments with a variety of health-care providers. Dr. Fitch is actively involved with a number of health-care trade associations, and is a frequent contributor to professional journals. Shortly after forming his consulting practice, he added a Ph.D. in organizational development to his B.A. and his Master of Arts degree in public administration.

Richard A. Keller, EMT-P, is an associate with Fitch & Associates and is recognized nationally as a leading expert in EMS reimbursement and operations. Mr. Keller has conducted extensive original research on new technologies for EMS and is the author of the 1987 National EMS Salary Survey published by *JEMS, the Journal of Emergency Medical Services*. He has served in operations management positions in EMS systems, developed the paramedic training program for Missouri Southern State College, and was instrumental in developing an EMS management information and accounts-receivables software system marketed nationally. Mr. Keller earned his Bachelor of Science degree in mathematics.

Doug Raynor, Ph.D., is director of management development at New York University Medical Center where he has implemented management training programs involving more than 3,000 health-care managers. In addition, Dr. Raynor is a member of the board of directors of Fitch & Associates and is heavily involved in the National EMS Management Academy sponsored annually by the firm. He has consulted with a number of major health-care institutions, centering on helping leaders meet the growing challenge of staff motivation and retention. He is the author of *Beyond Management* and *Coping Successfully*.

Christine M. Zalar, R.N., is an associate of Fitch & Associates, Inc. Her professional experience spans a wide spectrum of prehospital care including managing aeromedical and ground service and directing hospital emergency-care systems. As a consultant, Ms. Zalar has been responsible for developing multi-jurisidictional and multi-institutional programs for EMS providers. She is a recognized expert in rural emergency medical services and is active in many professional organizations. She recently added a Master of Arts Degree in psychology to her Bachelor of Science in nursing.

Fitch & Associates, Inc. is a health-care consulting firm with special emphasis on EMS. The group has consulted with more than 100 organizations in the United States and Canada, including state and local government, hospitals, volunteer services and private corporations. The firm is headquartered at 6812 Tower Drive, Kansas City, Missouri 64151; (816) 741-4422.